TYPE 2 DIABETES COOKBOOK FOR BEGINNERS:

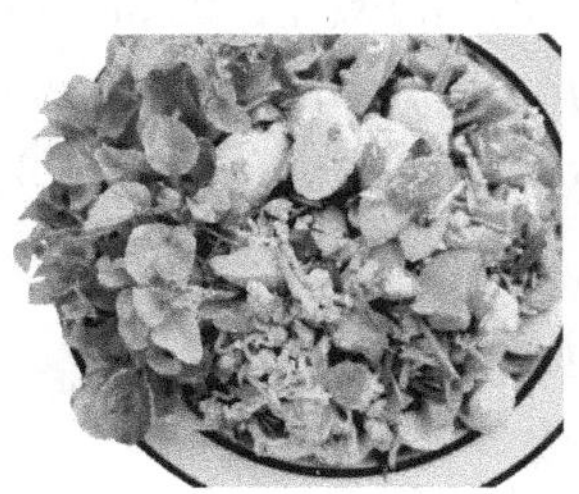

1100 Days of Super Easy, Tasty Low Sugar And Low Carb Recipes to Nourish and Manage High Blood Sugar Levels

Kimberly Mullins

Dear readers, as I reflect on the creation of this cookbook, my heart swells with gratitude for your unwavering support and dedication to learning more about type 2 diabetes. Your willingness to explore this topic means the world to me, as it highlights a shared commitment to understanding and managing this condition together. Thank you for investing your time and trust in these pages. May the knowledge within empower you on your health journey and bring newfound hope and confidence. With deep appreciation and warmest regards, [Kimberly Mullins].

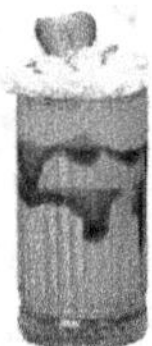

Disclaimer:

The information provided in this communication is for general informational
 only. It should not be considered as professional, legal, medical, or financial advice.
You are encouraged to seek advice and confirmation from qualified experts or
professionals before making any decisions or taking actions based on the content
provided here. We do not guarantee the accuracy, completeness, or suitability of the
information and shall not be liable for any errors, omissions, or damages arising from
its use. Any reliance you place on this information is strictly at your own risk. This
communication does not create a professional-client relationship. Any views or
opinions expressed here are solely those of the individual author and do not
necessarily represent the views of any organization or entity. We reserve the right to
modify, update, or remove content at any time without notice. By continuing to read
or interact with this content, you agree to these terms and conditions.

ABOUT THE AUTHOR

Kimberly Mullins is a renowned chef and dedicated dietitian with a passion for promoting healthy eating and lifestyle choices. With a culinary flair and a deep understanding of nutrition, she has made it her mission to inspire individuals and families to lead happier, healthier lives through the food they consume.

As a chef, Kimberly's expertise lies in crafting delectable dishes that not only tantalize the taste buds but also nourish the body. Her culinary creations seamlessly blend flavors, textures, and ingredients to make wholesome meals that cater to a wide range of dietary preferences and restrictions.

Simultaneously, Kimberly's background as a dietitian empowers her to provide sound nutritional advice and guidance. She understands the intricate relationship between food and well-being and strives to educate others on making informed choices for optimal health.

Beyond her professional pursuits, Kimberly is a loving wife and a devoted mother of two. Her own family serves as the cornerstone of her commitment to health and wellness, driving her to explore creative ways to make nutritious eating an enjoyable and integral part of daily life.

Kimberly Mullins' journey in the culinary and dietary world has led her to become a trusted source of expertise, helping countless individuals and families embrace a lifestyle that prioritizes health, balance, and deliciousness. Through her writing and culinary creations, she continues to inspire and guide others toward a more vibrant and wholesome way of living.

TABLE OF CONTENTS

INTRODUCTION

This is the "Type 2 Diabetes Cookbook for Beginners:" where the road to better health commences with taking one bite. Sometime back, an individual became a changed person – sick with type 2 diabetes. It was like a bolt from the blue on a fine day that sent their world into chaos. How could a person who thought they were healthy be handed such a huge responsibility?

However, they did not want to become victims of diabetes as many do. They made up their minds never to let this condition rule their lives. Full of determination and strongly supported by relatives and friends, they began looking for ways in which they could find out more about themselves and get healed from it. They held on to a craving for enlightenment as well as an unhesitating acceptance of change when stepping into the sphere of controlling diabetes.

That way some obstacles appeared before them, but it made them stronger than ever before. Occasionally, there were doubts concerning getting through as well as moments when everything seemed quite hopeless; however each barrier made them more resilient and indomitable than ever before. Navigating through grocery store aisles became easier for them because now they confidently selected foods that would nourish their bodies while stabilizing blood sugar levels.

Also, new cooking methods together with other recipes allowed them to realize how much they loved cooking. This was followed by great joy at mastering the art of turning common ingredients into delicious meals imbued with rich flavors that not only tickled the taste buds but also matched their health objectives

Significance of food in the prevention of type 2 diabetes

The significance of food in the prevention of type 2 diabetes should not be exaggerated. Diet plays a leading role in the development and management of this chronic ailment, thereby making it vital to understand how dietary choices may either exacerbate or alleviate its risk. This is a comprehensive overview of why food matters when it comes to thwarting type 2 diabetes:

1. Glycemic Impact: What we eat has the potential to affect our blood sugar levels directly. When broken down through digestion, carbohydrates mainly contribute towards this effect as they become glucose. High-carbohydrate diets, especially those with a high glycemic index, can cause rapid increases in blood sugars resulting in insulin resistance and type 2 diabetes mellitus (T2DM). Conversely, picking complex carbohydrates such as whole grains, legumes, and non-starchy vegetables that have low glycemic indices can help keep one's blood sugars stable hence minimizing the chances of developing diabetes.

2. Effect on Insulin Resistance: Insulin is a hormone produced by the pancreas that helps regulate blood sugar levels by facilitating the uptake of glucose into cells.When cells lose their sensitivity to insulin, they develop resistance against it thus causing elevated plasma glucose levels.Foods rich in saturated fats and refined sugars for instance are known culprits for insulin resistance which leads to the occurrence of T2DM. Conversely, a diet rich in fiber, healthy fats, and antioxidants can improve insulin sensitivity and lower the risk of diabetes.

3. Role in Weight Management: Excess fat, mostly abdominal, is a crucial determiner of the onset of type II diabetes mellitus. The amount and types of food we consume affect our weight and body composition directly. A diet rich in processed foods, sugary drinks and unhealthy fats can increase the risk of obesity and subsequent diabetes. Conversely, a diet high in whole grains, lean proteins, vegetables and fruits will facilitate weight loss hence minimizing chances of getting diabetes.

4. Nutrient Density and Disease Prevention: Nutrient dense meals supply important vitamins, minerals and antioxidants that promote general fitness reducing risks for long term conditions such as Type II Diabetes Mellitus (DM). Foods like fruits and vegetables, nuts and seeds have plenty of essential nutrients that support good health inhibiting insulin resistance thus inflammation – major causes of DM.

5. Long-Term Health Benefits: In addition to lowering the chances of contracting Type 2 Diabetes Mellitus; a healthy lifestyle has several other advantages. Plant-based diets enriched with lean proteins as well as unsaturated fats helps to reduce blood pressure levels, enhance lipid profiles by cholesterol reduction, decrease inflammation; all these benefit the cardiovascular system.

UNDERSTANDING TYPE 2 DIABETES

What is Type 2 Diabetes?

Type 2 diabetes is a chronic metabolic disorder characterized by high blood sugar levels (hyperglycemia) resulting from insulin resistance and inadequate insulin production. Insulin is a hormone produced by the pancreas that regulates blood sugar levels by facilitating the uptake of glucose into cells for energy. Elevated blood sugar levels are caused by cells that develop resistance to the actions of insulin in type 2 diabetes.

Symptoms and Warning Signs

Type 2 diabetes symptoms might differ from person to person and may appear gradually over time. Common symptoms and warning signs include:

1. Increased thirst and frequent urination: Excess glucose in the bloodstream leads to increased urine production, causing frequent urination. This, in turn, can result in dehydration and increased thirst.

2. Fatigue: Inadequate glucose uptake by cells can lead to fatigue and low energy levels.

3. Blurred vision: High blood sugar levels can cause changes in the shape of the lens in the eye, leading to blurred vision.

4. Slow wound healing: Elevated blood sugar levels can impair the body's ability to heal wounds and injuries.

5. Increased hunger: Despite eating regularly, individuals with type 2 diabetes may experience persistent hunger due to the body's inability to effectively utilize glucose for energy.

6. Unexplained weight loss: Some individuals with type 2 diabetes may experience unexplained weight loss despite an increased appetite. This is due to the body's inability to properly metabolize glucose and use it for energy.

Risk Factors and Causes

Several factors contribute to the development of type 2 diabetes, including:

1. Obesity and Sedentary Lifestyle: Excess body weight, particularly around the abdomen, increases the risk of insulin resistance and type 2 diabetes. The risk is significantly increased by inactivity and sedentary behavior.

2. Genetics: Family history and genetic predisposition play a significant role in the development of type 2 diabetes. Individuals with a family history of diabetes are at higher risk of developing the condition themselves.

3. Age: After the age of 45, in particular, there is an increased risk of type 2 diabetes. However, the condition is increasingly diagnosed in younger individuals due to rising rates of obesity and sedentary lifestyles.

4. Ethnicity: Certain ethnic groups, including African Americans, Hispanic/Latino Americans, Native Americans, Asian Americans, and Pacific Islanders, are at higher risk of developing type 2 diabetes.

5. Gestational Diabetes: Women who have experienced gestational diabetes during pregnancy are at increased risk of developing type 2 diabetes later in life.

The exact cause of type 2 diabetes is multifactorial and involves a combination of genetic, environmental, and lifestyle factors. Insulin resistance, where cells fail to respond adequately to insulin, is a key underlying mechanism in the development of the condition.

Untreated or poorly managed type 2 diabetes can lead to a range of serious complications, including:

1. Cardiovascular Disease: Individuals with diabetes are at increased risk of heart disease, stroke, and peripheral artery disease due to elevated blood sugar levels, high blood pressure, and abnormal cholesterol levels.

2. Kidney Damage (Nephropathy): Diabetes can damage the kidneys over time, leading to impaired kidney function and an increased risk of kidney failure.

3. Nerve Damage (Neuropathy): Elevated blood sugar levels can cause nerve damage, leading to symptoms such as numbness, tingling, and pain, particularly in the hands and feet.

4. Eye Problems (Retinopathy): Diabetes can damage the blood vessels in the retina, leading to vision problems and, in severe cases, blindness.

5. Foot Complications: Nerve damage and poor circulation in the feet increase the risk of foot ulcers, infections, and, in severe cases, amputation.

6. Skin Conditions: Individuals with diabetes are at increased risk of skin infections, particularly fungal and bacterial infections, due to impaired wound healing and compromised immune function.

7. Alzheimer's Disease: Some research suggests a link between type 2 diabetes and an increased risk of Alzheimer's disease and other forms of dementia.

Understanding Carbohydrates, Proteins, Fats, and Fiber

Carbohydrates

Along with proteins and lipids, carbohydrates are one of the three macronutrients that are necessary for human nutrition. They serve as the primary source of energy for the body, providing fuel for cellular functions, physical activity, and vital organ systems. Carbohydrates are composed of carbon, hydrogen, and oxygen atoms, with the basic building blocks being sugar molecules.

• **Types of Carbohydrates:**

1. **Simple Carbohydrates**: These are composed of one or two sugar molecules and are quickly digested and absorbed into the bloodstream, leading to rapid spikes in blood sugar levels. Common sources of simple carbohydrates include table sugar (sucrose), honey, fruit juices, candies, and sweets. While simple carbohydrates can provide quick energy, they are often devoid of essential nutrients and may contribute to fluctuations in blood sugar levels, making them less ideal for individuals with diabetes.

2. **Complex Carbohydrates:** These consist of longer chains of sugar molecules and take longer to digest, providing sustained energy and a more gradual rise in blood sugar levels. Complex carbohydrates are found in whole, unprocessed foods such as whole grains (e.g., brown rice, quinoa, oats), legumes (e.g., beans, lentils), vegetables (e.g., broccoli, spinach, sweet potatoes), and starchy foods (e.g., potatoes, corn). Unlike simple carbohydrates, complex carbohydrates are rich in fiber, vitamins, minerals, and phytonutrients, making them a healthier choice for individuals with diabetes.

• **Functions of Carbohydrates:**

1. **Energy Production:** Carbohydrates are converted into glucose during digestion, which serves as the primary fuel for cells, particularly in the brain and muscles. Glucose is transported through the bloodstream to cells throughout the body, where it is used for energy production through a process called cellular respiration. Adequate

intake of carbohydrates is essential for maintaining optimal energy levels, supporting physical activity, and preventing fatigue.

2. Glycogen Storage: Excess glucose that is not immediately needed for energy is converted into glycogen and stored in the liver and muscles for future use. Glycogen serves as a readily available source of glucose during periods of fasting or increased energy demand, such as prolonged exercise or periods of fasting. Maintaining adequate glycogen stores is essential for regulating blood sugar levels and preventing hypoglycemia (low blood sugar).

3. Dietary Fiber: Certain carbohydrates, known as dietary fiber, are indigestible by the body's enzymes and pass through the digestive tract relatively unchanged. Fiber adds bulk to stool, promotes bowel regularity, and helps prevent constipation. Additionally, soluble fiber, found in foods like oats, legumes, and fruits, can help lower cholesterol levels and improve blood sugar control by slowing down the absorption of glucose in the bloodstream.

• <u>**Carbohydrates and Diabetes Management:**</u>

For individuals with diabetes, understanding how carbohydrates affect blood sugar levels is crucial for managing their condition effectively. Carbohydrate-containing foods have the most significant impact on blood sugar levels, as they are broken down into glucose during digestion. Therefore, monitoring carbohydrate intake and making wise food choices are essential strategies for diabetes management.

1. Carbohydrate counting is a common method used by individuals with diabetes to manage their blood sugar levels. It involves calculating the total grams of carbohydrates in a meal or snack and adjusting insulin doses or medication accordingly. This approach allows individuals to make informed decisions about portion sizes and food choices while maintaining stable blood sugar levels throughout the day.

2. The glycemic index (GI) is a scale that ranks carbohydrate-containing foods based on their effect on blood sugar levels. Foods with a high GI (e.g., white bread, sugary cereals, white rice) cause a rapid increase in blood sugar levels, while those with a low GI (e.g., whole grains, legumes, non-starchy vegetables) lead to a slower and more gradual rise in blood sugar levels. Choosing foods with a lower GI can help individuals with diabetes better manage their blood sugar levels and improve overall glycemic control.

3. Controlling portion sizes of carbohydrate-containing foods is essential for preventing spikes in blood sugar levels. Measuring or estimating serving sizes, paying attention to food labels, and being mindful of carbohydrate content can help individuals with diabetes maintain stable blood sugar levels and achieve their dietary goals.

4. In addition to considering the quantity of carbohydrates consumed, it's also important to pay attention to the quality of carbohydrates. Choosing whole, minimally processed sources of carbohydrates, such as whole grains, fruits, vegetables, and legumes, can provide more nutrients, fiber, and slower-digesting carbohydrates compared to refined and processed carbohydrate sources like white bread, sugary snacks, and sweetened beverages. This can help individuals with diabetes better manage their blood sugar levels and improve overall health.

5. Regular monitoring of blood sugar levels is essential for individuals with diabetes to assess the impact of carbohydrate intake on their glycemic control. Testing blood sugar levels before and after meals can help identify how different foods and portion sizes affect blood sugar levels and guide adjustments in dietary choices and insulin doses as needed.

6. The timing of carbohydrate intake can also influence blood sugar levels. Spreading carbohydrate intake evenly throughout the day, rather than consuming large amounts of carbohydrates at once, can help prevent sharp spikes and drops in blood sugar levels. Additionally, consuming carbohydrates in combination with protein, fat, and fiber can help slow down the absorption of glucose and minimize fluctuations in blood sugar levels.

Protein

Protein is a crucial micronutrient essential for numerous bodily functions, including muscle repair and growth, hormone production, immune function, and enzyme activity. For individuals with diabetes, understanding the role of protein in the diet is essential for managing blood sugar levels, supporting overall health, and preventing complications associated with the condition.

• <u>Types of Protein</u>

1. Complete Proteins: Complete proteins contain all nine essential amino acids required by the body. The body is unable to produce certain amino acids, hence it must get them from food. Animal-based foods such as meat, poultry, fish, eggs, and dairy products are complete sources of protein, providing a full complement of essential amino acids necessary for optimal health.

2. Incomplete Proteins: Incomplete proteins lack one or more essential amino acids and are typically found in plant-based sources such as beans, lentils, nuts, seeds, and grains. While individual plant-based foods may not contain all essential amino acids, combining complementary sources of protein, such as beans and rice or hummus and whole grain pita bread, can provide a complete array of amino acids necessary for supporting bodily functions.

• <u>Functions of Protein</u>

1. Protein is essential for repairing and building muscle tissue, especially after physical activity or injury. Adequate protein intake supports muscle maintenance and growth, which is particularly important for individuals with diabetes to support metabolic health and prevent muscle wasting.

2. Many hormones, including insulin, are composed of proteins or amino acids. Insulin, in particular, plays a central role in regulating blood sugar levels by facilitating the uptake of glucose into cells for energy production. Consuming adequate protein supports insulin production and function, which is crucial for managing diabetes effectively.

3. Proteins are integral components of the immune system, playing a vital role in the production of antibodies that defend the body against infections and diseases. Adequate protein intake supports immune function, helping individuals with diabetes to prevent and fight off infections, which can be more common in this population due to compromised immune function.

• <u>Protein and Diabetes Management</u>

Understanding how protein affects blood sugar levels and incorporating protein-rich foods into the diet can help individuals with diabetes manage their condition more effectively.

1. Blood Sugar Control: Unlike carbohydrates, protein has a minimal impact on blood sugar levels when consumed in moderation. However, excessive protein intake can lead to gluconeogenesis, a process in which the liver converts protein into glucose, potentially raising blood sugar levels. Therefore, it's essential for individuals with diabetes to balance protein intake with carbohydrate intake and monitor blood sugar levels accordingly.

2. Satiety and Weight Management : Protein-rich foods are often more filling and satisfying than carbohydrate-rich foods, leading to reduced hunger and calorie intake. Including protein at meals and snacks can help individuals with diabetes feel fuller for longer, preventing overeating and supporting weight management efforts, which are important for managing blood sugar levels and preventing obesity-related complications.

3. Muscle Health: Maintaining muscle mass is important for individuals with diabetes to support metabolic health and prevent insulin resistance. Consuming adequate protein, especially from high-quality sources such as lean meats, poultry, fish, tofu, and legumes, can help preserve muscle mass and promote overall well-being.

• <u>Incorporating Protein into the Diet</u>

1. Choose Lean Protein Sources: Opt for lean cuts of meat, poultry without skin, fish, seafood, and low-fat dairy products to minimize intake of saturated fat and cholesterol. Plant-based protein sources such as beans, lentils, tofu, tempeh, and edamame are also excellent options for individuals looking to reduce their consumption of animal products.

2. Include Protein at Every Meal: Incorporate protein-rich foods into each meal and snack to help balance blood sugar levels and promote satiety. Aim to include a variety of protein sources in your diet to ensure a diverse array of amino acids and nutrients.

3. Monitor Portion Sizes: Pay attention to portion sizes when consuming protein-rich foods, as excessive intake can lead to excess calorie consumption and weight gain. Aim for a palm-sized portion of protein at each meal, along with plenty of non-starchy vegetables, whole grains, and healthy fats.

4. Consider Timing: Distribute protein intake evenly throughout the day, rather than consuming large amounts of protein at once, to support muscle repair and growth and optimize blood sugar control.

5. **Protein's Effect on Glucose Levels** Although protein has a minimal direct impact on blood glucose levels, it can still affect glycemic control indirectly. Consuming protein alongside carbohydrates can slow down the digestion and absorption of carbohydrates, leading to a more gradual rise in blood glucose levels after meals. This can be particularly beneficial for individuals with diabetes in managing postprandial blood sugar spikes.

6. Protein Quality: In addition to quantity, the quality of protein is important for overall health. High-quality protein sources provide essential amino acids in optimal ratios and are often associated with additional nutrients. Because they contain all of the essential amino acid profiles, animal-based proteins such lean meats, poultry, fish, and eggs are regarded as high-quality proteins. Plant-based proteins, while generally lower in one or more essential amino acids, can still be part of a healthy diet when consumed in combination to provide a full range of amino acids.

7. Potential Risks of High-Protein Diets: While protein is essential for health, consuming excessive amounts of protein, especially from animal sources, may pose certain risks. High-protein diets can increase the workload on the kidneys and may be associated with an increased risk of kidney disease, particularly in individuals with pre-existing kidney conditions. Additionally, some research suggests that a high intake of red and processed meats may be linked to an increased risk of certain health conditions, including heart disease and certain types of cancer.

Fats

Fats are a vital component of the diet, serving as a concentrated source of energy and playing critical roles in various bodily functions. For individuals with diabetes, comprehending the nuances of fats is essential for optimizing blood sugar control, managing weight, and reducing the risk of cardiovascular complications. Let's delve into the intricacies of fats, exploring their types, functions, and implications for diabetes management.

• **Types of Fats**

1. Saturated Fats: Saturated fats are predominantly found in animal products such as red meat, poultry, full-fat dairy, and butter. They are also present in certain plant-based sources like coconut oil and palm oil. Consuming high amounts of saturated fats has been linked to elevated LDL cholesterol levels and an increased risk of heart disease, a significant concern for individuals with diabetes who are already predisposed to cardiovascular complications.

2. Trans Fats: Trans fats are artificially produced through hydrogenation, a process that converts liquid vegetable oils into solid fats to enhance shelf life and texture in processed foods. Common sources of trans fats include margarine, fried foods, baked goods, and packaged snacks. Trans fats raise LDL cholesterol levels while lowering HDL (good) cholesterol levels, contributing to a higher risk of heart disease. It's crucial for individuals with diabetes to minimize their intake of trans fats to protect their cardiovascular health.

3. Monounsaturated Fats: Monounsaturated fats are liquid at room temperature and are abundant in foods such as olive oil, avocados, nuts, and seeds. They have been associated with improved lipid profiles, including lower LDL cholesterol levels and higher HDL cholesterol levels. Incorporating monounsaturated fats into the diet can promote heart health and help manage diabetes by supporting better blood sugar control and reducing inflammation.

4. Polyunsaturated Fats: Polyunsaturated fats include omega-3 and Omega-6 fatty acids, both of which are essential for health but must be obtained from dietary sources since the body cannot produce them. Omega-3 fatty acids are found in fatty fish (e.g., salmon, mackerel, sardines), flaxseeds, chia seeds, and walnuts, and are known for their anti-inflammatory properties and cardiovascular benefits. Omega-6 fatty acids are prevalent in vegetable oils (e.g., soybean oil, corn oil, sunflower oil) and are necessary for various bodily functions but should be consumed in moderation to keep the ratio of omega-3 fatty acids in check

• **<u>Functions of Fats</u>**

1. Fats serve as the body's primary long-term energy storage mechanism, providing a concentrated source of energy that can be utilized during periods of fasting or sustained physical activity. For individuals with diabetes, optimizing fat metabolism can help stabilize blood sugar levels and prevent energy dips between meals.

2. Fats are integral components of cell membranes, contributing to membrane integrity, flexibility, and fluidity. They also play a role in cell signaling, gene expression, and the transport of fat-soluble vitamins (A, D, E, K). Maintaining optimal fat intake is essential for supporting cellular health and overall physiological function, including insulin sensitivity and glucose metabolism.

3. Fats are precursors to hormone synthesis, including steroid hormones such as cortisol, estrogen, and testosterone. Hormones play critical roles in regulating metabolism, inflammation, stress response, and reproductive function. Maintaining adequate fat intake is necessary for hormone production and balance, which can influence blood sugar regulation and overall health in individuals with diabetes.

• **<u>Implications for Diabetes Management</u>**

1. Cardiovascular Health: Heart disease is a leading cause of morbidity and mortality in individuals with diabetes. Therefore, managing fat intake, particularly saturated and trans fats, is crucial for reducing the risk of cardiovascular complications. Choosing heart-healthy fats, such as monounsaturated and polyunsaturated fats, over less healthy options can help lower LDL cholesterol levels, improve HDL cholesterol levels, and reduce the risk of heart disease.

2. Blood Sugar Control: While fats do not directly impact blood sugar levels, they can influence insulin sensitivity and glucose metabolism. Consuming excessive amounts of saturated and trans fats may impair insulin action and contribute to insulin resistance, a key factor in the development and progression of type 2 diabetes. Therefore, replacing unhealthy fats with healthier alternatives can support better blood sugar control and metabolic health.

3. Weight Management: Fats are calorie-dense, providing nine calories per gram compared to four calories per gram for carbohydrates and proteins. Consuming too many calories from fat can contribute to weight gain and obesity, both of which are risk factors for type 2 diabetes and its complications. Therefore, monitoring portion sizes and choosing healthier fats can help individuals with diabetes manage their weight and prevent obesity-related complications.

5. Portion Control: While healthy fats are an essential part of a balanced diet, it's crucial to consume them in moderation. Even healthy fats, when consumed in excess, can contribute to weight gain and other health issues. Portion control is key to managing fat intake and supporting overall health, particularly for individuals with diabetes who may be at increased risk of obesity and its associated complications.

6. Cooking Methods: The way fats are prepared and cooked can impact their health effects. Opting for healthier cooking methods such as baking, grilling, steaming, or sautéing with small amounts of oil can help minimize the addition of extra fats and calories to meals. Avoiding deep-frying and excessive use of oil in cooking can help reduce the intake of unhealthy fats and promote heart health.

7. Reading Food Labels: Understanding how to interpret food labels can help individuals with diabetes make informed choices about the fats they consume. Pay attention to the type and amount of fats listed on food labels, aiming to choose products that are low in saturated and trans fats and high in healthier fats like monounsaturated and polyunsaturated fats. Be wary of hidden sources of unhealthy fats in processed and packaged foods.

Fiber

Plant-based meals contain fiber, a kind of carbohydrate that the human body is unable to absorb. While it does not contribute calories or raise blood sugar levels, fiber plays a crucial role in promoting overall health, particularly for individuals with diabetes. Understanding the different types of fiber, their health benefits, and how to incorporate them into the diet is essential for managing blood sugar levels, supporting digestive health, and reducing the risk of chronic diseases.

• Types of Fiber

1. Soluble Fiber: Soluble fiber dissolves in water to form a gel-like substance in the digestive tract. This type of fiber helps slow down the absorption of glucose into the bloodstream, leading to more stable blood sugar levels after meals. Soluble fiber also binds to cholesterol in the digestive tract, helping to lower LDL (bad) cholesterol levels and reduce the risk of heart disease. Good sources of soluble fiber include oats, barley, legumes (beans, peas, lentils), fruits (apples, oranges, berries), and vegetables (carrots, Brussels sprouts, broccoli).

2. Insoluble Fiber: Insoluble fiber does not dissolve in water and adds bulk to stool, promoting regular bowel movements and preventing constipation. While insoluble fiber does not directly affect blood sugar levels, it plays a crucial role in digestive health by keeping the digestive system moving smoothly. Whole grains (whole wheat, brown rice, quinoa), nuts, seeds, and the skins of fruits and vegetables are rich sources of insoluble fiber.

• Health Benefits of Fiber

1. Blood Sugar Control: Soluble fiber helps slow down the absorption of carbohydrates, preventing rapid spikes in blood sugar levels after meals. This can be particularly beneficial for individuals with diabetes in managing postprandial blood glucose levels and reducing the risk of hyperglycemia (high blood sugar). Consuming a diet high in fiber can also improve insulin sensitivity and reduce the need for insulin or other diabetes medications.

2. Cholesterol Reduction: Soluble fiber binds to cholesterol in the digestive tract, preventing its absorption into the bloodstream and promoting its excretion. Regular consumption of soluble fiber-rich foods can help lower LDL cholesterol levels and reduce the risk of heart disease, which is especially important for individuals with diabetes who are at increased risk of cardiovascular complications.

3. Weight Management: High-fiber foods are often lower in calories and more filling than low-fiber foods, leading to reduced hunger and calorie intake. By promoting satiety and reducing overeating, fiber can help support weight management efforts, which is important for individuals with diabetes in managing blood sugar levels and preventing obesity-related complications.

4. Digestive Health: Insoluble fiber adds bulk to stool and promotes regular bowel movements, preventing constipation and reducing the risk of digestive disorders such as diverticulosis and hemorrhoids. Additionally, fiber helps maintain a healthy balance of gut bacteria, which is important for overall digestive health and immune function.

• <u>Incorporating Fiber into the Diet</u>

1. Increase Consumption of Whole Plant Foods: Whole plant foods, such as fruits, vegetables, whole grains, legumes, nuts, and seeds, are naturally rich sources of fiber. Incorporating a variety of these foods into the diet can help ensure an adequate intake of both soluble and insoluble fiber.

2. Choose Whole Grains: Opt for whole grains such as whole wheat, brown rice, quinoa, oats, and barley instead of refined grains, which have had the bran and germ removed, stripping them of their fiber and nutrient content.

3. Eat Plenty of Fruits and Vegetables: Aim to fill half your plate with fruits and vegetables at each meal, as these foods are rich in fiber, vitamins, minerals, and antioxidants. Choose a variety of colorful fruits and vegetables to ensure a diverse range of nutrients and fiber types.

4. Include Legumes in Your Diet: Legumes, including beans, peas, lentils, and chickpeas, are excellent sources of both soluble and insoluble fiber, as well as protein and other essential nutrients. Add legumes to soups, salads, stir-fries, and casseroles for a fiber-rich boost.

5. Read Food Labels: When purchasing packaged foods, such as breakfast cereals, granola bars, and snack foods, check the nutrition label for fiber content. Look for products that contain at least 3-5 grams of fiber per serving to ensure an adequate intake of fiber.

6. Increase Fiber Intake: Gradually To prevent digestive discomfort such as bloating, gas, and cramping, increase your fiber intake gradually and drink plenty of water to help fiber move smoothly through the digestive tract.

7. Impact on Blood Glucose Monitoring: While fiber itself does not significantly raise blood sugar levels, some individuals with diabetes may experience delayed effects on blood glucose levels after consuming high-fiber meals. It's essential for individuals monitoring their blood sugar to be aware of these potential delayed effects and adjust their insulin or medication doses accordingly. Regular monitoring and tracking of blood sugar levels before and after meals containing high-fiber foods can help individuals understand their individual responses and optimize their diabetes management strategies.

8. Hydration: Increasing fiber intake should be accompanied by adequate hydration to prevent constipation and support optimal digestive function. Fiber absorbs water in the digestive tract, softening stool and promoting regular bowel movements. Therefore, individuals with diabetes should aim to drink plenty of water throughout the day, especially when consuming high-fiber foods, to ensure proper hydration and optimal digestive health.

9. Potential for Gas and Bloating: Some high-fiber foods, particularly those rich in certain types of fibers such as oligosaccharides found in beans and cruciferous vegetables, may cause gas and bloating in some individuals. While these symptoms are usually temporary and subside as the body adjusts to increased fiber intake, it's essential for individuals with diabetes to be mindful of their tolerance to high-fiber foods and make adjustments as needed to minimize discomfort while still incorporating fiber-rich foods into their diet.

10. Individualized Approach: While increasing fiber intake is generally beneficial for individuals with diabetes, it's essential to recognize that individual responses to dietary fiber may vary. Factors such as gastrointestinal sensitivity, medication use, and overall dietary patterns can influence how the body responds to increased fiber intake.

Foods to Include in Your Diet

1. Fruits and Vegetables

Arrange a vibrant assortment of fruits and vegetables on your platter. These nutrient-rich foods are packed with vitamins, minerals, fiber, and antioxidants that support overall health and reduce the risk of chronic diseases like diabetes, heart disease, and cancer. Aim to include a variety of fruits and vegetables in your diet, incorporating different colors and types to ensure you're getting a wide range of nutrients.

2. Whole Grains

Choose whole grains over refined grains to reap the benefits of fiber, vitamins, and minerals. Whole grains such as oats, brown rice, quinoa, barley, and whole wheat provide sustained energy, promote satiety, and support digestive health. Incorporate whole grains into your meals and snacks to boost nutrient intake and support overall well-being.

3. Lean Proteins

Include lean protein sources in your diet to support muscle health, promote satiety, and stabilize blood sugar levels. Opt for options such as poultry, fish, tofu, tempeh, beans, lentils, and low-fat dairy products. These protein-rich foods provide essential amino acids and nutrients without excess saturated fat and calories.

4. Healthy Fats

Don't shy away from healthy fats, as they play a crucial role in supporting heart health, brain function, and hormone production. Choose sources of unsaturated fats such as avocados, nuts, seeds, olive oil, and fatty fish. These fats supply the body with necessary fatty acids and aid in lowering inflammation

5. Dairy or Dairy Alternatives

Incorporate dairy products or dairy alternatives into your diet to meet your calcium and vitamin D needs. Choose low-fat or fat-free options such as milk, yogurt, and cheese, or opt for plant-based alternatives like almond milk, soy milk, and coconut yogurt. These calcium-rich foods support bone health and provide essential nutrients for overall well-being.

Foods to Limit or Avoid

1. Processed and Sugary Foods

Minimize your intake of processed and sugary foods, including sugary snacks, candies, desserts, pastries, and sweetened beverages. These foods are high in added sugars, refined carbohydrates, and unhealthy fats, which can contribute to weight gain, insulin resistance, and chronic diseases.

2. Saturated and Trans Fats

Limit your consumption of foods high in saturated and trans fats, such as fried foods, fatty meats, butter, margarine, and processed snacks. These fats can cause inflammation in the body, raise cholesterol, and raise the risk of heart disease. Opt for healthier fats from sources like nuts, seeds, avocados, and olive oil instead.

3. High-Sodium Foods

Reduce your intake of high-sodium foods such as processed meats, canned soups, salty snacks, and fast food. Excess sodium can lead to high blood pressure, fluid retention, and cardiovascular problems. Choose low-sodium options and flavor your foods with herbs, spices, and citrus instead of salt.

4. Alcohol

Limit your alcohol consumption to moderate levels, as excessive drinking can have negative effects on health. Alcohol provides empty calories, can contribute to weight gain, and may increase the risk of chronic diseases like liver disease, heart disease, and certain cancers. Stick to recommended guidelines for alcohol consumption and enjoy in moderation.

5. Artificial Sweeteners and Additives

Be cautious of artificial sweeteners and additives found in processed foods and beverages. While they may provide sweetness without calories, some research suggests they may have negative effects on metabolism and gut health. Choose whole, minimally processed foods whenever possible and read labels carefully to avoid unnecessary additives.

Grocery Shopping and Pantry Essentials

Healthy grocery shopping is not just about filling your cart with nutritious foods; it's also about making smart choices, staying within your budget, and navigating the aisles with confidence. I'm here to provide you with some practical tips to help you make the most of your next trip to the grocery store:

1. Plan Ahead

Before heading to the store, take some time to plan your meals for the week. Make a list of the ingredients you'll need for each meal, along with any snacks or staples you're running low on. Planning ahead can help you stay focused and avoid impulse purchases.

2. Shop the Perimeter

When you arrive at the store, start by shopping the perimeter. This is where you'll find fresh produce, lean proteins, dairy products, and whole grains. Fill your cart with plenty of fruits and vegetables, lean meats, fish, poultry, eggs, low-fat dairy, and whole grain bread and pasta.

3. Read Labels Carefully

As you shop, be sure to read food labels carefully. Take note of ingredient lists, portion sizes, and nutritional information. Look for products that are low in added sugars, saturated fats, and sodium, and high in fiber, vitamins, and minerals.

4. Choose Whole Foods

Whenever possible, choose whole, minimally processed foods. These foods are typically higher in nutrients and lower in added sugars, unhealthy fats, and preservatives. Instead of reaching for pre-packaged snacks and meals, consider making your own with fresh, wholesome ingredients.

5. Stock Up on Staples

Don't forget to stock up on pantry staples like beans, lentils, rice, quinoa, oats, nuts, seeds, and spices. These versatile ingredients can be used to create a variety of healthy meals and snacks, and they tend to have a longer shelf life.

6. Limit Packaged and Processed Foods

While it's okay to include some packaged and processed foods in your diet, try to limit them as much as possible. These foods are often high in added sugars, unhealthy fats, and sodium, and they may lack essential nutrients. Instead, focus on whole, nutrient-rich foods that nourish your body and support your health.

7. Don't Shop Hungry

Avoid shopping on an empty stomach, as this can lead to impulse purchases and unhealthy food choices. Eat a balanced meal or snack before heading to the store to help curb cravings and stay on track with your healthy eating goals.

8. Stay Hydrated

Don't forget to drink plenty of water while you shop. Staying hydrated can help you make better food choices, keep your energy levels up, and prevent dehydration. Consider bringing a reusable water bottle with you to sip on as you browse the aisles.

9. Compare Prices and Brands

To get the most for your money, take the time to compare products and prices. Consider buying generic or store-brand products, which are often cheaper than name brands but just as nutritious. Look for sales, coupons, and discounts to save even more on your grocery bill.

10. Be Flexible

Finally, be flexible with your shopping list and willing to make substitutions based on what's available and in season. Embrace variety and try new foods and recipes to keep your meals interesting and your taste buds happy.

1. Whole Grains
  - Brown rice
  - Quinoa
  - Whole wheat pasta
  - Whole grain bread
  - Oats (steel-cut or rolled)

2. Beans and Legumes
  - Black beans
  - Chickpeas
  - Lentils
  - Kidney beans
  - Pinto beans

3. Nuts and Seeds
  - Almonds
  - Walnuts
  - Chia seeds
  - Flaxseeds
  - Pumpkin seeds

4. Lean Proteins
  - Skinless poultry (chicken, turkey)
  - Fish (salmon, tuna, trout)
  - Tofu
  - Tempeh
  - Lean beef or pork portions

5. Fresh Produce
  - Cruciferous vegetables (broccoli, cauliflower, Brussels sprouts)
  - Leafy greens (spinach, kale, Swiss chard
  - Colorful vegetables (bell peppers, carrots, tomatoes)
  - Berries (blueberries, strawberries, raspberries)
  - Citrus fruits (oranges, grapefruits, lemons)

6. Healthy Fats

  - Extra virgin olive oil
  - Avocado
- Fatty fish (salmon, mackerel, sardines)

7. Low-Sodium Seasonings and Flavorings
  - Herbs (rosemary, thyme, basil, oregano)
  - Spices (cinnamon, turmeric, ginger, garlic powder)
  - Vinegars (balsamic vinegar, apple cider vinegar)
  - Low-sodium soy sauce or tamari

8. Low-Sugar Condiments and Sauces
  - Choose tomato sauce that doesn't have any added sugars.
  - Mustard
  - Hot sauce
  - Salsa (choose varieties with no added sugars)
  - Low-sugar salad dressings

9. Sugar Substitutes
  - Stevia
  - Monk fruit
  - Erythritol

11. Dairy or Dairy Alternatives
  - Low-fat or fat-free milk
  - Almond milk without sugar or other plant-based milk substitutes
  - Plain Greek yogurt (unsweetened)
  - Cottage cheese (low-fat or fat-free)

12. Whole Grain Snacks
  - Whole grain crackers
  - Air-popped popcorn
  - Whole grain cereal (look for options with no added sugars)

13. High-Fiber Cereals and Bran
  - High-fiber cereal (look for options with at least 5 grams of fiber per serving)
  - Wheat bran
  - Psyllium husk

14. Low-Sodium Broths and Stocks
  - Low-sodium vegetable broth

- Low-sodium chicken or beef broth
- Low-sodium bouillon cubes or granules

15. Canned or Jarred Goods
  - Canned tomatoes (no added sugars)
  - Canned beans (rinsed and drained to reduce sodium)
  - Jarred roasted red peppers
  - Canned tuna or salmon (packed in water)

16. Whole Grain Flour and Baking Ingredients
  - Whole wheat flour
  - Almond flour
  - Coconut flour
  - Baking powder
  - Baking soda

17. Low-Sodium Condiments
  - Low-sodium ketchup
  - Reduced-sodium soy sauce or tamari
  - Low-sodium Worcestershire sauce
  - Dijon mustard (unsweetened)

18. Herbal Teas and Infusions
  - Green tea
  - Herbal teas (peppermint, chamomile, ginger)
  - Rooibos tea

19. Cooking Oils and Vinegars
  - Canola oil
  - Grapeseed oil
  - White vinegar
  - Balsamic vinegar (no added sugars)

20. Frozen Fruits and Vegetables
  - Frozen berries
  - Frozen mixed vegetables
  - Frozen spinach or kale
  - Frozen cauliflower rice

Reading Food Labels

1. The serving size is your guiding star on the food label. It tells you the amount of food considered a single serving and helps you interpret the rest of the nutritional information accurately.

2. Keep an eagle eye on total carbohydrates, including sugars and fiber. As they impact blood sugar levels the most, understanding their content can empower you to make informed choices. Opt for foods lower in carbohydrates to maintain stable blood sugar levels.

3. Fiber is your ally in diabetes management. It slows down carbohydrate absorption, aiding in blood sugar control. Load up on fiber-rich foods like whole grains, fruits, vegetables, legumes, and nuts for sustained energy and digestive health.

4. Added sugars can sneak into unsuspecting foods, wreaking havoc on blood sugar levels. Be vigilant and opt for foods with minimal added sugars or natural sweeteners like stevia and monk fruit.

5. While fats don't directly impact blood sugar, they play a vital role in heart health and weight management. Choose foods low in saturated and trans fats and rich in unsaturated fats to support overall well-being.

6. Keep an eye on sodium content, especially if you're at risk of cardiovascular complications. Limit high-sodium foods and opt for low-sodium alternatives to protect your heart health.

7. Take a peek at the ingredient list to understand what's really in your food. Ingredients are listed in descending order by weight, so if unhealthy ingredients like sugar or hydrogenated oils appear near the top, consider opting for a healthier alternative.

8. Don't overlook the "% Daily Value" (%DV) column on food labels. This percentage tells you how much of a particular nutrient one serving of the food contributes to your daily recommended intake. Aim for foods that provide lower percentages of saturated

fat, sodium, and added sugars, while aiming for higher percentages of fiber, vitamins, and minerals.

9. Keep an eye out for sneaky sources of added sugars that may not be obvious. Ingredients like high-fructose corn syrup, cane sugar, and syrups (e.g., malt syrup, rice syrup) can contribute to hidden sugars in processed foods. Be vigilant and opt for products with minimal added sugars or those sweetened with natural alternatives.

10. Be cautious of health claims and buzzwords on food packaging, such as "low-fat," "sugar-free," or "all-natural." While these labels may sound enticing, they don't always indicate a healthier choice. Turn the package around and scrutinize the nutrition label and ingredient list to make a truly informed decision about the product's nutritional value.

Portion Control

1. Visual cues are your best friends when estimating portion sizes. Imagine your palm for proteins, your fist for carbohydrates, and your thumb for fats to guide your choices.

2. When dining out, study the menu like a pro. Look for healthier preparation methods and balanced options, and don't hesitate to customize your order to suit your needs.

3. Split meals with a companion to manage portion sizes and calorie intake effectively. If splitting isn't an option, ask for a to-go box upfront and portion out a suitable serving size before diving in.

4. Tune in to your body's hunger and fullness cues, and savor each bite mindfully. Avoid distractions and eat slowly to prevent overeating and promote satisfaction.

5. Plan your meals and snacks ahead of time, and use tools like measuring cups and food scales to portion out foods accurately. This proactive approach sets you up for success in managing your diabetes.

6. Visualize your plate as a canvas for a balanced meal. Arrange your plate such that non-starchy vegetables make up half of it, lean protein makes up a quarter of it, and

whole grains or starchy veggies make up the other quarter. This simple strategy helps keep portions in check while ensuring a nutrient-rich meal.

7. Allow yourself time to adjust to smaller portion sizes. It's normal to experience initial hunger pangs or cravings as you transition, but with time, your body will adapt, and you'll find satisfaction in smaller, more nutrient-dense meals.

8. Take a proactive approach to meal planning by incorporating a variety of nutrient-dense foods into your daily meals and snacks. Prioritize whole, minimally processed foods rich in vitamins, minerals, fiber, and protein to nourish your body and support optimal health.

9. Explore healthier alternatives to your favorite foods to reduce calorie and carbohydrate intake without sacrificing flavor or satisfaction. For example, swap white rice for cauliflower rice, soda for sparkling water with lemon or cucumber, or potato chips for air-popped popcorn seasoned with herbs and spices.

10. Tune in to your body's hunger and fullness signals to guide your eating patterns. Eat when you're physically hungry and stop when you're comfortably satisfied, rather than eating out of habit or in response to external cues like stress or boredom. Learning to differentiate between physical hunger and emotional hunger is key to developing a healthy relationship with food.

MEAL PLANNING

Meal planning is a valuable tool for anyone, especially those looking to prevent or manage type 2 diabetes. It involves deciding in advance what meals you'll eat for a certain period, typically a week, and then preparing for those meals by creating a shopping list, buying ingredients, and possibly prepping some components ahead of time. Here's a breakdown of the meal planning process:

Before you start meal planning, it's essential to set goals related to your health, dietary preferences, and lifestyle. Consider factors such as your calorie and nutrient needs, any dietary restrictions or preferences you have, and your schedule. This will help you tailor your meal plan to meet your specific needs and preferences. Once you've established your goals and preferences, start selecting recipes and meals for the week. Look for recipes that align with your dietary goals and include a balance of carbohydrates, protein, and healthy fats. Choose meals that you enjoy and that are easy to prepare, especially if you have a busy schedule.

Based on the recipes and meals you've chosen, create a shopping list of all the ingredients you'll need for the week. Organize your list by food categories (e.g., produce, proteins, grains) to make shopping more efficient. Be sure to check your pantry and fridge for any ingredients you already have on hand to avoid purchasing duplicates. Once you have your shopping list prepared, head to the grocery store to purchase your ingredients. Stick to your list as much as possible to avoid impulse purchases and stay within your budget. Consider shopping at local markets or farmers' markets for fresh, seasonal produce and supporting small businesses in your community. To streamline meal preparation during the week, consider prepping some ingredients ahead of time. This could include washing and chopping vegetables, marinating meats, cooking grains or beans, or assembling freezer-friendly meals. By prepping ingredients in advance, you can save time and make cooking during the week more manageable.

Throughout the week, use your meal plan and prepped ingredients to prepare meals according to your schedule. Be flexible and make adjustments as needed based on your preferences and any changes in your plans. Remember to savor your meals and enjoy the process of nourishing your body with delicious, homemade food. After the week is over, take some time to reflect on your meal plan and how it worked for you. Consider what went well and what could be improved, and make adjustments as needed for future meal plans. Over time, you'll become more adept at meal planning and find a routine that works best for you.

28 DAY MEAL PLAN

Week 1

DAY 1
Breakfast: Curry-Avocado Crispy Egg Toast
Lunch: Salmon salad with white beans
Dinner: Shrimp with Green Beans

DAY 2
Breakfast: Vegetarian Egg and Lentils on Toast
Lunch: Stuffed potato with salsa and beans
Dinner: Sole with parsley and mint

DAY 3
Breakfast: Mushroom freezer Breakfast Burritos
Lunch: Keto Sushi
Dinner: Cauliflower potato salad

DAY 4
Breakfast: Tomato and Egg stacks
Lunch: Turkey and cheddar lettuce wraps
Dinner: Cauliflower Tacos

DAY 5
Breakfast: Sweet potato Blueberry Sausage frittata
Lunch: Lean pork and veggie tacos or quesadillas
Dinner: Chicken pasta and spinach soup

DAY 6
Breakfast: Turkish Egg with Greek yogurt
Lunch: Low sodium bean soup and a cheese stick with sunflower seeds
Dinner: Spinach and black bean burritos

DAY 7
Breakfast: Veggie loaded Chickpea waffles

Lunch: Sweet potato bowl with black bean and quinoa tofu stir fry
Dinner: Sesame garlic beef and broccoli with whole wheat noodles

<u>Week 2</u>

DAY 8
Breakfast: White Cheddar Zucchini Muffins
Lunch: Turkey patties with avocado
Dinner: Chicken meatballs with whipped tahini and arugula

DAY 9
Breakfast: Mini corn, cheese and Basil Frittatas
Lunch: Lemony Chicken and rice soup
Dinner: Roasted garlic parmesan cabbage

DAY 10
Breakfast: Peaches and cream parfaits with maple syrup
Lunch: Salmon salad with white beans
Dinner: Balsamic butter chicken bites

DAY 11
Breakfast: Sweet Potato Blueberry Sausage Frittatas
Lunch:
Dinner: Barley and pumpkin beef stew

DAY 12
Breakfast: Curry-Avocado Crispy Egg Toast
Lunch: Keto sushi
Dinner: Hamburger steak with onions and gravy

DAY 13
Breakfast: Turkish Egg with Greek yogurt
Lunch: Spaghetti squash bolognese
Dinner: Kale, sausage and pepper pasta

DAY 14
Breakfast: Veggie loaded Chickpea waffles
Lunch: Turkey patties with avocado

Dinner: Barley and pumpkin beef stew

<u>Week 3</u>

DAY 15
Breakfast: Sweet potato Blueberry Sausage frittata
Lunch: Lean pork and veggie tacos or quesadillas
Dinner: Chicken pasta and spinach soup

DAY 16
Breakfast: Vegetarian Egg and Lentils on Toast
Lunch: Stuffed potato with salsa and beans
Dinner: Sole with parsley and mint

DAY 17
Breakfast: Mushroom freezer Breakfast Burritos
Lunch: Keto Sushi
Dinner: Cauliflower potato salad

DAY 18
Breakfast: Sweet potato Blueberry Sausage frittata
Lunch: Lean pork and veggie tacos or quesadillas
Dinner: Chicken pasta and spinach soup

DAY 19
Breakfast: Mini corn, cheese and Basil Frittatas
Lunch: Lemony Chicken and rice soup
Dinner: Roasted garlic parmesan cabbage

DAY 20
Breakfast: Peaches and cream parfaits with maple syrup
Lunch: Salmon salad with white beans
Dinner: Balsamic butter chicken bites

DAY 21
Breakfast: Curry-Avocado Crispy Egg Toast
Lunch: Salmon salad with white beans
Dinner: Shrimp with Green Beans

<u>Week 4</u>

DAY 22
Breakfast: Tomato and Egg stacks
Lunch: Turkey and cheddar lettuce wraps
Dinner: Cauliflower Tacos

DAY 23
Breakfast: White Cheddar Zucchini Muffins
Lunch: Turkey patties with avocado
Dinner: Chicken meatballs with whipped tahini and arugula

DAY 24
Breakfast: Sweet potato Blueberry Sausage frittata
Lunch: Lean pork and veggie tacos or quesadillas
Dinner: Chicken pasta and spinach soup

DAY 25
Breakfast: Curry-Avocado Crispy Egg Toast
Lunch: Keto sushi
Dinner: Hamburger steak with onions and gravy

DAY 26
Breakfast: Mini corn, cheese and Basil Frittatas
Lunch: Lemony Chicken and rice soup
Dinner: Roasted garlic parmesan cabbage

DAY 27
Breakfast: Curry-Avocado Crispy Egg Toast
Lunch: Salmon salad with white beans
Dinner: Shrimp with Green Beans

DAY 28
Breakfast: Peaches and cream parfaits with maple syrup
Lunch: Salmon salad with white beans
Dinner: Balsamic butter chicken bites

BREAKFAST RECIPES

Veggie-Loaded Chickpea Waffles

Prep Time: 15 minutes
Cook Time: 10 minutes
Servings: 4

Ingredients
- 1 cup chickpea flour
- 1 teaspoon baking powder
- 1/2 teaspoon baking soda
- 1/2 teaspoon salt
- 1/4 teaspoon black pepper
- 1/2 teaspoon garlic powder
- 1/2 teaspoon onion powder
- 1/2 cup grated zucchini
- 1/2 cup grated carrot
- 1/4 cup chopped spinach
- 2 green onions, finely chopped
- 2 tablespoons chopped fresh parsley
- 2 large eggs
- 1/4 cup almond milk, unsweetened (or any other type of milk)
- 2 tablespoons olive oil

Procedure
1. Preheat your waffle iron according to manufacturer instructions.

2. In a large mixing bowl, combine the chickpea flour, baking powder, baking soda, salt, black pepper, garlic powder, and onion powder. Stir until well combined. Add the grated zucchini, grated carrot, chopped spinach, chopped green onions, and chopped parsley to the dry ingredients. Mix until the vegetables are evenly distributed throughout the flour mixture.

3. To get the right consistency, you can add a bit of extra almond milk if the batter appears too thick. Pour the wet ingredients into the bowl with the dry ingredients and vegetable mixture. Stir until all the ingredients are fully incorporated and a thick batter forms. Evenly distribute the batter across the waffle iron's surface

4. Once the waffle iron is preheated, lightly grease it with cooking spray or a small amount of olive oil.

5. Spoon the batter onto the waffle iron, using about 1/2 cup of batter for each waffle. The batter should be spread evenly across the surface of the waffle iron. Close the waffle iron and cook the waffles according to the manufacturer instructions, until they are golden brown and crispy on the outside.

5. Carefully remove the cooked waffles from the waffle iron and transfer them to a plate. Serve the Veggie-Loaded Chickpea Waffles warm, topped with your favorite toppings such as Greek yogurt, salsa, avocado slices, or a drizzle of maple syrup.

Notes
• If you enjoy spicy flavors, consider adding a pinch of red pepper flakes or a dash of hot sauce to the waffle batter for a bit of extra kick.

• Don't be afraid to experiment with different herbs and spices to add flavor to the waffles. Try adding dried herbs like oregano, basil, or thyme, or spices like cumin or smoked paprika for a unique flavor profile.

• These waffles are perfect for meal prep! Once cooked, allow them to cool completely, then store them in an airtight container or resealable plastic bag in the freezer. When ready to eat, simply reheat them in the toaster or oven for a quick and convenient breakfast option.

• To make these waffles a more balanced meal, consider serving them with a source of protein such as scrambled eggs, Greek yogurt, or turkey sausage patties. This will help keep you feeling full and satisfied until your next meal.

Nutritional Information (per serving - 1 waffle)
- Calories: 210 kcal
- Protein: 10g
- Fat: 10g
- Carbohydrates: 21g

- Fiber: 5g
- Sugars: 3g

White Cheddar Zucchini Muffins

Prep Time: 15 minutes
Cook Time: 20 minutes
Servings: 12 muffins

Ingredients
- 1 1/2 cups grated zucchini (about 1 medium zucchini)
- 1 1/2 cups whole wheat flour
- 1 cup shredded white cheddar cheese
- 1/4 cup olive oil
- 1/4 cup unsweetened applesauce
- 1/4 cup plain Greek yogurt
- 2 large eggs
- 1/4 cup honey or maple syrup (optional, adjust to taste)
- 1 teaspoon baking powder
- 1/2 teaspoon baking soda
- 1/2 teaspoon salt
- 1/2 teaspoon onion powder
- ½ teaspoon garlic powder
- 1/4 teaspoon black pepper
- Cooking spray or muffin liners

Procedure
1. Preheat your oven to 350°F (175°C). Grease a 12-cup muffin tin with cooking spray or line with muffin liners.

2. Grate the zucchini using a box grater or food processor. After grating the zucchini, place it in a fresh kitchen towel and press off any extra moisture.

3.   In a large mixing bowl, combine the whole wheat flour, baking powder, baking soda, salt, garlic and onion powder, and black pepper. Stir until well combined.

4. In a separate bowl, whisk together the olive oil, unsweetened applesauce, Greek yogurt, eggs, and honey or maple syrup (if using) until smooth.

5. Pour the wet ingredients into the bowl of dry ingredients and mix until just combined. Be careful not to overmix.

6. Gently fold the grated zucchini and shredded white cheddar cheese into the muffin batter until evenly distributed.

7. Divide the batter evenly among the prepared muffin cups, filling each cup about 3/4 full.

8. When the muffins are golden brown and a toothpick inserted into the center comes out clean, remove the muffin tray from the oven and bake for another 18 to 20 minutes

9. Remove the muffins from the oven and allow them to cool in the muffin tin for a few minutes before transferring them to a wire rack to cool completely.

Nutritional Information (per serving)
- Calories: 160 kcal
- Protein: 5g
- Fat: 8g
- Carbohydrates: 17g
- Fiber: 2g
- Sugars: 4g

Turkish Eggs with Greek Yogurt

Prep Time: 5 minutes
Cook Time: 5 minutes
Servings: 2

Ingredients
- 4 large eggs
- 1 cup Greek yogurt
- 2 cloves garlic, minced
- 2 tablespoons olive oil
- 1 teaspoon paprika
- 1 teaspoon dried oregano
- ½ teaspoon Salt
- ¼ teaspoon pepper
Chopped fresh parsley or cilantro as a garnish; optionally add some heat with red pepper flakes

Procedure

1. In a medium-sized mixing bowl, combine the Greek yogurt, minced garlic, olive oil, paprika, dried oregano, salt, and pepper. Stir well to fully combine all of the ingredients. Set aside.

2. Fill a large saucepan with water, about 2-3 inches deep, and bring it to a gentle simmer over medium heat. In a small bowl or cup, crack each of the eggs. Carefully slide each egg into the simmering water. Use a spoon to gently shape the egg whites around the yolks.

3. Allow the eggs to poach for 3-4 minutes, or until the egg whites are set but the yolks are still runny. Using a slotted spoon, remove the poached eggs from the water and put them aside

4. Divide the Greek yogurt mixture evenly between two serving plates, spreading it out into a thin layer. Carefully place two poached eggs on top of the Greek yogurt mixture on each plate.

5. Sprinkle chopped parsley or cilantro over the eggs for garnish. If desired, add a sprinkle of red pepper flakes for extra heat. Serve the Turkish Eggs with Greek Yogurt immediately, while still warm.

<u>Notes</u>

• Feel free to adjust the seasoning of the Greek yogurt mixture to suit your taste preferences. You can add a squeeze of lemon juice for a tangy flavor or sprinkle in some smoked paprika for a smoky kick.

• Boost the nutritional content of the dish by adding finely chopped vegetables like tomatoes, cucumbers, or bell peppers to the Greek yogurt mixture. These additions will not only add flavor and texture but also provide additional vitamins and minerals.

• Get creative with the herbs used to garnish the dish. Try using fresh dill, basil, or mint in place of parsley or cilantro for a different flavor profile.

• To make the meal more filling and balanced, consider serving the Turkish Eggs with Greek Yogurt alongside whole grain bread or toast. This will provide additional fiber and complex carbohydrates to help keep you satisfied.

• For a vegan-friendly version of this recipe, you can substitute the eggs with pan-fried tofu or scrambled tofu seasoned with turmeric and black salt for an egg-like flavor. Use dairy-free yogurt made from coconut or almond milk in place of Greek yogurt.

Nutritional Information (per serving)
- Calories: 280 kcal
- Protein: 18g
- Fat: 20g
- Carbohydrates: 6g
- Fiber: 1g
- Sugars: 4g

Mini Corn, Cheese, and Basil Frittatas

Prep Time: 15 minutes
Cook Time: 20 minutes
Servings: 6 mini frittatas

Ingredients
- 4 large eggs
- 1/4 cup unsweetened almond milk (or any milk of your choice)
- 1/2 cup canned corn kernels, drained
- 1/4 cup shredded low-fat cheddar cheese

- 2 tablespoons chopped fresh basil leaves
- 1/4 teaspoon garlic powder
- 1/4 teaspoon onion powder
- Salt and pepper to taste
- Cooking spray or olive oil

Procedure

1. Preheat your oven to 375°F (190°C). Grease a 6-cup muffin tin with cooking spray or lightly coat with olive oil.

2. In a mixing bowl, whisk together the eggs, unsweetened almond milk, garlic powder, onion powder, salt, and pepper until well combined.

3. Stir in the drained corn kernels, shredded low-fat cheddar cheese, and chopped fresh basil leaves into the egg mixture, ensuring they are evenly distributed.

4. Pour the egg mixture evenly into the prepared muffin tin, filling each cup about 3/4 full.

5. Place the muffin tin in the preheated oven and bake for 18-20 minutes, or until the frittatas are set and lightly golden brown on top.

6. Remove the muffin tin from the oven and allow the frittatas to cool for a few minutes before carefully removing them from the tin using a spoon or spatula.
    - Serve warm at room temperature.

<u>Notes</u>

• Feel free to customize the fillings based on your preferences or what you have on hand. You can substitute the corn with other vegetables like diced bell peppers, spinach, or mushrooms. You can also experiment with different types of cheese, such as feta or mozzarella.

• While basil adds a fresh and aromatic flavor to the frittatas, you can also use other herbs like parsley, chives, or cilantro. If using dried herbs, reduce the amount by half, as dried herbs are more potent than fresh.

• These mini frittatas are perfect for meal prep. You can bake a batch ahead of time and store them in the refrigerator for up to 3-4 days. Simply reheat them in the microwave or toaster oven before serving.

• To make a complete meal, consider serving the frittatas with a side salad, whole grain bread, or roasted potatoes. Adding additional fiber-rich foods will help balance the meal and keep you feeling full and satisfied.

Nutritional Information (per serving - 1 mini frittata)
- Calories: 90 kcal
- Protein: 7g
- Fat: 5g
- Carbohydrates: 5g
- Fiber: 1g
- Sugars: 1g

Mushroom Freezer Breakfast Burritos

Prep Time: 20 minutes
Cook Time: 20 minutes
Servings: 6 breakfast burritos

Ingredients
- 6 large whole wheat or low-carb tortillas
- 6 large eggs
- 1/2 cup diced bell peppers (any color)
- 1/2 cup diced onions
- 1 cup diced tomatoes
- 1 cup diced cooked turkey sausage (or any lean protein of your choice)
- 1 cup shredded low-fat cheddar cheese
- 1 tablespoon olive oil
- Salt and pepper to taste
- Cooking spray

Procedure
1. Dice the bell peppers, onions, tomatoes, and cooked turkey sausage into small, bite-sized pieces.

2. In a large skillet, heat olive oil over medium heat. In a bowl, whisk the eggs until well beaten. Season with salt and pepper to taste. Pour the beaten eggs into the skillet and scramble until cooked through. Remove from heat and set aside.

3. In the same skillet, add a little more olive oil if needed. Add the diced bell peppers and onions to the skillet and sauté until softened, about 3-4 minutes. Add the diced tomatoes to the skillet and cook for an additional 2-3 minutes until softened.

4. Lay out the tortillas on a clean surface. Divide the scrambled eggs, sautéed vegetables, cooked turkey sausage, and shredded cheese evenly among the tortillas, placing the fillings in the center of each tortilla.

5. Fold the sides of each tortilla inward, then roll them up tightly from the bottom to create a burrito shape.

6. Wrap each assembled burrito individually in aluminum foil or plastic wrap. Place the wrapped burritos in a resealable plastic bag or airtight container and store them in the freezer.

7. To serve, just zap them in the toaster oven or microwave. Microwave on high for 2-3 minutes, or until heated through. Serve warm either on their own or with a side of salsa, avocado, or Greek yogurt for dipping.

<u>Notes</u>
• Feel free to customize the fillings based on your preferences or dietary needs. You can add or substitute ingredients like spinach, black beans, avocado, or salsa for added flavor and nutrients.

• These breakfast burritos are perfect for meal prep. You can assemble a batch ahead of time and store them in the freezer for a quick and convenient breakfast option throughout the week. Simply reheat them in the microwave or oven when ready to eat.

• To help with portion control and manage blood sugar levels, consider using smaller tortillas or reducing the amount of filling in each burrito. You can also serve them with a side of fresh fruit or Greek yogurt to round out the meal.

• Store the assembled burritos in airtight containers or resealable plastic bags to prevent freezer burn and maintain freshness. Label the containers with the date and contents for easy identification.

Nutritional Information (per serving - 1 breakfast burrito)
- Calories: 290 kcal
- Protein: 19g
- Fat: 12g
- Carbohydrates: 25g
- Fiber: 4g
- Sugars: 3g

Vegetarian Eggs and Lentils on Toast

Prep Time: 10 minutes
Cook Time: 20 minutes
Servings: 2

Ingredients
- 1/2 cup dry green or brown lentils
- 4 slices whole grain bread
- 4 large eggs
- 1/4 cup crumbled feta cheese
- 1/4 cup diced tomatoes
- Half a cup of chopped bell peppers, any color
- Cooking spray or olive oil
- Salt and pepper to taste
- Fresh parsley or cilantro for garnish (optional)

Procedure

1. After rinsing with cold water, drain the lentils. The lentils and 1 1/2 cups of water should be combined in a medium pot and brought to a boil. Lower the heat to a simmer, cover, and let the lentils cook for 15 to 20 minutes, or until they are soft but not falling apart. After cooking, remove any leftover water and reserve.

2. While the lentils are cooking, toast the whole grain bread slices until golden brown and crisp. Set aside.

3. In a non-stick skillet, heat cooking spray or olive oil over medium heat. Crack the eggs into the skillet and cook to your desired level of doneness. For sunny-side-up eggs, cook until the whites are set but the yolks are still runny. For scrambled eggs, whisk the eggs in a bowl before adding them to the skillet and cook until they are scrambled and cooked through.

4. Divide the cooked lentils evenly between the toasted bread slices, spreading them out in an even layer. Top each slice of toast and lentils with cooked eggs. Sprinkle diced tomatoes, diced bell peppers, and crumbled feta cheese over the eggs. Season with salt and pepper to taste..

Notes
• Enhance the flavor of the lentils and eggs by incorporating herbs and spices such as garlic powder, onion powder, cumin, or smoked paprika. You can sprinkle these seasonings over the lentils or eggs while cooking for added depth of flavor.

• Boost the nutritional value of this dish by adding leafy greens such as spinach or kale. Simply wilt the greens in the skillet with the eggs or add them directly to the lentils while they're cooking. Leafy greens are rich in vitamins, minerals, and antioxidants, making them an excellent addition to any meal.

• While feta cheese adds a tangy flavor to the dish, feel free to experiment with different types of cheese such as goat cheese, grated Parmesan, or shredded mozzarella. Choose low-fat or reduced-fat cheese options to keep the saturated fat content in check.

• Elevate the flavor profile of the dish by drizzling it with a healthy sauce or dressing. Consider topping the eggs and lentils with a dollop of Greek yogurt, a homemade salsa or avocado mash, or a drizzle of balsamic glaze. These additions not only add flavor but also provide additional nutrients and creaminess to the dish.

• Pair with a side salad made with mixed greens, chopped vegetables, and a light vinaigrette dressing. The salad adds freshness and crunch to the meal while providing extra fiber and micronutrients.

Nutritional Information (per serving)
- Calories: 340 kcal
- Protein: 22g

- Fat: 12g
- Carbohydrates: 36g
- Fiber: 11g
- Sugars: 5g

Whole-Grain Cereal with Ground Flaxseed, Egg, and Oatmeal

Prep Time: 5 minutes
Cook Time: 10 minutes
Servings: 1

Ingredients
- 1/4 cup old-fashioned oats
- 1/2 cup water or milk of your choice (unsweetened almond milk, skim milk, etc.)
- 1 large egg
- 1 tablespoon ground flaxseed
- 1/4 teaspoon cinnamon (optional)
- 1/2 tablespoon honey or maple syrup (optional, for sweetness)
- Fresh berries or sliced fruit for topping (optional)

Procedure
1. In a small saucepan, bring the water or milk to a boil over medium heat. Stir in the old-fashioned oats and reduce the heat to low. Simmer the oats, stirring occasionally, for 5-7 minutes or until the oatmeal is thickened and creamy.

2. While the oatmeal is cooking, prepare the egg. You can either poach, fry, or scramble the egg according to your preference.

If poaching: Bring a pot of water to a gentle simmer. Crack the egg into a small bowl, then carefully slide it into the simmering water. Cook for about 3-4 minutes until the egg whites are set but the yolk is still runny.

If frying or scrambling: Heat a non-stick skillet over medium heat and coat with cooking spray or a small amount of olive oil. Crack the egg into the skillet and cook to your desired level of doneness.

3. Once the oatmeal is cooked, transfer it to a serving bowl. Sprinkle ground flaxseed and cinnamon (if using) over the oatmeal and stir to combine. Drizzle honey or maple syrup (if using) over the oatmeal for added sweetness, if desired. Place the cooked egg on top of the oatmeal.

4. Garnish with fresh berries or sliced fruit for added flavor and nutrients, if desired.

<u>Notes</u>
• Consider adding other nutritious ingredients to the oatmeal for additional flavor and health benefits. You can stir in a tablespoon of almond butter or peanut butter for added protein and healthy fats. Alternatively, add a tablespoon of chia seeds or hemp seeds for extra fiber and omega-3 fatty acids.

• Customize your cereal bowl with a variety of toppings to suit your taste preferences. Sliced bananas, diced apples, chopped nuts, or dried fruit like raisins or cranberries are all excellent options. These toppings add sweetness, texture, and additional nutrients to the dish.

• Feel free to experiment with different spices to enhance the flavor of the oatmeal. Try adding a pinch of nutmeg, ginger, or cardamom for a warm and aromatic twist. You can also sprinkle a teaspoon of cocoa powder for a hint of chocolate flavor without adding extra sugar.

• If you prefer a sweeter cereal bowl, opt for natural sweeteners like mashed ripe banana or unsweetened applesauce instead of honey or maple syrup. These alternatives offer sweetness without raising blood sugar levels.

• Serve the cereal bowl with a side of Greek yogurt, cottage cheese, or a handful of nuts for added protein and satiety.

Nutritional Information (per serving)
- Calories: 310 kcal
- Protein: 17g
- Fat: 13g
- Carbohydrates: 33g
- Fiber: 6g

- Sugars: 9g

Curry-Avocado Crispy Egg Toast

Prep Time: 10 minutes
Cook Time: 15 minutes
Servings: 2

Ingredients
- 4 slices whole grain bread
- 2 large eggs
- 1 ripe avocado
- 1 tablespoon curry powder
- 1/4 teaspoon garlic powder
- 1/4 teaspoon onion powder
- 1/4 teaspoon ground turmeric
- Salt and pepper to taste
- Cooking spray or olive oil

Procedure
1. Preheat your oven to 375°F (190°C). After halving the avocado and removing the pit, transfer the flesh to a small bowl.

Mash the avocado with a fork until smooth. Stir in the curry powder, garlic powder, onion powder, ground turmeric, salt, and pepper until well combined. Set aside.

2. Place the slices of whole grain bread on a baking sheet. Brush the bread lightly with olive oil. Toast the bread in the preheated oven for 5-7 minutes, or until golden and crispy.

3. While the bread is toasting, heat a non-stick skillet over medium heat. Lightly coat the skillet with cooking spray or a small amount of olive oil. Crack the eggs into the skillet and cook to your desired level of doneness. For crispy edges, allow the eggs to cook undisturbed for a few minutes until the edges are golden brown and crispy.

4. Spread a generous amount of the curry-avocado mixture onto each slice of toasted bread. Place a crispy fried egg on top of the avocado spread.

5. Serve immediately while still warm. Optionally, garnish with additional curry powder or fresh herbs like cilantro or parsley for added flavor and presentation.

Notes

• If you enjoy spicy flavors, consider adding a pinch of red pepper flakes or a dash of hot sauce to the avocado spread for some added heat.

• To elevate the flavor and texture of the dish, consider adding fresh ingredients such as sliced tomatoes, cucumber, or red onion as additional toppings for the toast.

• Feel free to customize the spice blend to suit your taste preferences. You can experiment with different spices such as cumin, paprika, or garam masala to create a unique flavor profile for the avocado spread.

• For a creamier texture, you can blend the avocado mixture with a splash of lemon juice or Greek yogurt before spreading it onto the toast. This will add a tangy flavor and smooth consistency to the spread.

• To make it a complete meal, consider serving the Curry-Avocado Crispy Egg Toast with a side salad made with mixed greens, diced vegetables, and a light vinaigrette dressing. The salad adds freshness and additional nutrients to the dish.

Nutritional Information (per serving)
- Calories: 290 kcal
- Protein: 12g
- Fat: 15g
- Carbohydrates: 28g
- Fiber: 8g
- Sugars: 2g

Tomato and Egg Stacks

Prep Time: 10 minutes

Cook Time: 15 minutes

Servings: 2

Ingredients
- 2 large tomatoes
- 4 large eggs
- 1/2 cup baby spinach leaves
- 1/4 cup crumbled feta cheese
- 2 tablespoons chopped fresh basil
- Salt and pepper to taste
- Olive oil or cooking spray

Procedure

1. Preheat your oven to 375°F (190°C). Slice the tomatoes horizontally into thick slices, about 1/2 inch thick. Crack each egg into a small bowl or cup, being careful not to break the yolks. Wash the baby spinach leaves and chop the fresh basil.

2. Lightly grease a baking sheet with olive oil or cooking spray. Place half of the tomato slices on the baking sheet, leaving space between each slice. Layer each tomato slice with a handful of baby spinach leaves, followed by a sprinkle of crumbled feta cheese and chopped basil. Carefully place the remaining tomato slices on top of the spinach, cheese, and basal layers to create stacks.

3. Create a small well in the center of each tomato stack using the back of a spoon. Carefully pour one egg into each well, ensuring that the yolk remains intact. Add salt and pepper to the eggs.

4. Place the baking sheet in the preheated oven and bake for 12-15 minutes, or until the egg whites are set and the yolks are still slightly runny.

5. Once cooked, remove from the oven. Use a spatula to carefully transfer each stack to a serving plate. Serve the stacks immediately, garnished with additional chopped basil if desired.

Notes
• If you enjoy spicy flavors, consider sprinkling some red pepper flakes or adding a dash of hot sauce to the Tomato and Egg Stacks before serving. This will add a kick of heat and extra flavor to the dish.

• Feel free to customize the filling ingredients based on your preferences and dietary needs. You can add ingredients like diced bell peppers, sliced mushrooms, or cooked crumbled turkey sausage for added flavor and texture.

• For an extra boost of healthy fats and creaminess, consider adding sliced avocado on top before serving. Avocado adds richness and nutritional benefits to the dish.

• To make the meal more filling and balanced, consider serving the Tomato and Egg Stacks with a side of whole grain toast or whole wheat English muffins. This will add fiber and complex carbohydrates to help keep you satisfied.

• If you're lactose intolerant or following a dairy-free diet, you can omit the feta cheese or replace it with a dairy-free cheese alternative. You can also skip the cheese altogether and add extra herbs and seasonings for flavor.

Nutritional Information (per serving)
- Calories: 180 kcal
- Protein: 13g
- Fat: 11g
- Carbohydrates: 7g
- Fiber: 2g
- Sugars: 4g

Peaches & Cream Parfaits with Maple Bacon Crumbles

Prep Time: 15 minutes
Cook Time: 15 minutes
Servings: 2

<u>For the Maple Bacon Crumbles</u>
- 2 slices of bacon
- 1 tablespoon maple syrup

For the Parfaits
- 2 ripe peaches, diced
- 1 cup Greek yogurt (unsweetened)
- 2 tablespoons honey or maple syrup
- 1/4 cup granola (unsweetened)
- Fresh mint leaves for garnish (optional)

Procedure
1. Preheat your oven to 400°F (200°C).
Arrange the bacon pieces on a parchment paper-lined baking sheet.
Drizzle the bacon slices with maple syrup. Bake in the preheated oven for 10-15 minutes, or until the bacon is crispy and caramelized.

2. Remove the bacon from the oven and let it cool. After the bacon has cooled, break it into small pieces and save.

3. In two serving glasses or bowls, layer half of the diced peaches at the bottom of each glass. Next, add a layer of Greek yogurt on top of the peaches, followed by a drizzle of honey or maple syrup.

4. Next, add a layer of Greek yogurt on top of the peaches, followed by a drizzle of honey or maple syrup. Place granola on top of the yogurt mixture in a layer.. Repeat the layers until the glasses are filled, ending with a layer of granola on top.

5. Top each parfait with a sprinkle of the maple bacon crumbles. Garnish the Peaches & Cream Parfaits with fresh mint leaves, if desired.

Notes
• For extra crunch and texture, consider adding chopped nuts such as almonds, walnuts, or pecans to the parfait layers. Toasted coconut flakes or seeds like pumpkin or sunflower seeds can also be a delicious addition.

• While peaches are delicious in this recipe, feel free to experiment with other fruits such as strawberries, blueberries, or raspberries. You can use fresh or frozen fruit depending on availability and personal preference.

• If you follow a vegan diet, you can easily make this recipe vegan-friendly by using plant-based yogurt (such as almond or coconut yogurt) instead of Greek yogurt. Additionally, you can replace the bacon with coconut bacon or omit it altogether.

• Instead of using honey or maple syrup to sweeten the parfaits, you can opt for natural sweeteners like mashed ripe bananas, date syrup, or agave nectar. These alternatives add sweetness without the need for refined sugars.

• Enhance the flavor of the parfaits by incorporating ingredients like cinnamon, vanilla extract, or a sprinkle of nutmeg. These spices can add warmth and depth to the dish, complementing the sweetness of the fruit and yogurt.

Nutritional Information (per serving)
- Calories: 280 kcal
- Protein: 15g
- Fat: 8g
- Carbohydrates: 40g
- Fiber: 4g
- Sugars: 28g

Sweet Potato Blueberry Sausage Frittata

Prep Time: 15 minutes
Cook Time: 25 minutes
Servings: 4

Ingredients
- One medium sweet potato, cut into dice and peel
- 4 chicken sausages, sliced
- 1 cup fresh blueberries
- 6 large eggs
- 1/4 cup milk (unsweetened almond milk or any milk of your choice)
- 1/2 teaspoon dried thyme
- Salt and pepper to taste

- One tablespoon of cooking spray or olive oil

Procedure
1.   Preheat your oven to 375°F (190°C). In a saucepan, warm the olive oil over medium heat. Add the diced sweet potatoes to the skillet and cook for 5-7 minutes, or until they are tender and lightly browned.

2. Remove the cooked sweet potatoes from the skillet and set aside. In the same skillet, add the sliced chicken sausages and cook for 3-4 minutes, or until they are browned and cooked through. The cooked sausages should be taken out of the skillet and placed aside.

3.   In a large mixing bowl, whisk together the eggs, milk, dried thyme, salt, and pepper until well combined. Grease a 9-inch pie dish or oven-safe skillet with olive oil or cooking spray.

4. Spread the cooked sweet potatoes and chicken sausages evenly in the bottom of the pie dish. Scatter the fresh blueberries over the sweet potatoes and sausages. Pour the egg mixture evenly over the ingredients in the pie dish.

5. Place the pie dish in the preheated oven and bake for 15-20 minutes, or until the frittata is set in the center and lightly golden on top.

6. Once cooked, remove from the oven and let it cool for a few minutes. Slice the frittata into wedges and serve warm.

<u>Notes</u>
• Boost the nutritional value of the frittata by adding a handful of fresh spinach or kale to the egg mixture before baking. These leafy greens will add extra fiber, vitamins, and minerals to the dish.

• The cooked sausages should be taken out of the skillet and placed asideYou can opt for turkey or pork sausage instead of chicken sausage, or choose a vegetarian or plant-based sausage for a meatless option.

• While blueberries add a delicious sweetness to the frittata, you can experiment with other types of fruits as well. Consider using diced apples, pears, or even sliced strawberries for a different flavor profile.

• If you enjoy cheese, consider sprinkling some grated cheese over the top of the frittata before baking. Sharp cheddar, feta, or goat cheese would all pair well with the flavors of the sweet potatoes, blueberries, and sausage.

• This frittata is perfect for meal prep! It may be prepared in advance and kept for up to three or four days in the refrigerator. Simply reheat individual slices in the microwave or enjoy them cold for a quick and convenient meal option.

• For a complete meal, consider serving the Sweet Potato Blueberry Sausage Frittata with a side salad, whole grain toast, or roasted vegetables. This will add variety to the meal and help balance out the flavors and nutrients.

Nutritional Information (per serving)
- Calories: 260 kcal
- Protein: 18g
- Fat: 14g
- Carbohydrates: 15g
- Fiber: 3g
- Sugars: 6g

BEVERAGE, DRINK, SMOOTHIE AND JUICE RECIPES

Strawberry and Orange Rhubarb Refresher with Mint

Prep Time: 10 minutes
Cook Time: 10 minutes
Chilling Time: 2 hours
Servings: 4

Ingredients

-Two cups freshly chopped, one-inch-long chunks of rhubarb
- 1 cup fresh strawberries, hulled and sliced
- 1 orange, juiced
- 1/4 cup granulated sweetener of your choice, such as stevia or erythritol
- 2 cups water
- Several fresh mint leaves, plus additional for decoration
- Ice cubes

Procedure

1. Wash and chop the rhubarb into 1-inch pieces. Hull and slice the strawberries. Juice the orange.

2. In a medium saucepan, combine the chopped rhubarb, sliced strawberries, orange juice, granulated sweetener, and water. After setting the pot on medium heat, bring the contents to a boil. Once the rhubarb is soft and tender, reduce the heat to low and simmer the mixture for around 10 minutes

3. Remove the saucepan from the heat and add a handful of fresh mint leaves to the rhubarb mixture. Let the mixture cool to room temperature to allow the flavors to meld together.

4. Once cooled, strain the rhubarb mixture through a fine mesh sieve or cheesecloth to remove any pulp or seeds. Transfer the strained liquid to a pitcher and refrigerate it for at least 2 hours, or until well chilled.

5. To serve, fill glasses with ice cubes. Pour the chilled Strawberry and Orange Rhubarb Refresher into the glasses.
   - Garnish each glass with a sprig of fresh mint leaves for added freshness and aroma. Stir before drinking

Nutritional Information
- Per serving (1/4 of the recipe): Calories: 30 kcal, Carbohydrates: 8g, Protein: 1g, Fat: 0g, Saturated Fat: 0g, Cholesterol: 0mg, Sodium: 5mg, Fiber: 2g, Sugar: 4g

Vanilla Chai Coffee Cooler

Prep Time: 5 minutes
Cook Time: 5 minutes
Chilling Time: 2 hours
Servings: 2

Ingredients
- 1 cup of room temperature coffee after it has been brewed
- 1 cup unsweetened almond milk (or any unsweetened milk of your choice)
- 1 chai tea bag
- 1 teaspoon pure vanilla extract
- 1 tablespoon granulated sweetener of your choice, such as stevia or erythritol
- Ice cubes
- Whipped cream and ground cinnamon for garnish (optional)

Procedure

1. Brew 1 cup of coffee and let it cool to room temperature. In a small saucepan, heat the unsweetened almond milk over medium heat until it begins to simmer. Remove from heat.

2. Add the chai tea bag to the hot almond milk and let it steep for 3-5 minutes to infuse the milk with chai flavor. Remove the tea bag and discard it.

3. In a pitcher or large glass, combine the cooled brewed coffee, chai-infused almond milk, pure vanilla extract, and granulated sweetener. Stir well to combine.

4. Place the pitcher or glass in the refrigerator and chill the mixture for at least 2 hours, or until well chilled.

5. Once chilled, pour the Vanilla Chai Coffee Cooler into glasses filled with ice cubes. Optionally, top each glass with a dollop of whipped cream and a sprinkle of ground cinnamon for garnish.

Nutritional Information

- *Per serving (1/2 of the recipe, without optional toppings):* Calories: 30 kcal, Carbohydrates: 2g, Protein: 1g, Fat: 1g, Saturated Fat: 0g, Cholesterol: 0mg, Sodium: 80mg, Fiber: 0g, Sugar: 0g

Pumpkin Eggnog

Prep Time: 10 minutes
Cook Time: 10 minutes
Chilling Time: 2 hours
Servings: 4

Ingredients

- 2 cups unsweetened almond milk (or any unsweetened milk of your choice)
- 1/2 cup canned pumpkin puree
- 2 large eggs

- 2 tablespoons granulated sweetener of your choice, such as stevia or erythritol
- 1 teaspoon pure vanilla extract
- 1/2 teaspoon ground cinnamon
- 1/4 teaspoon ground nutmeg
- 1/4 teaspoon ground ginger
- Pinch of ground cloves
- Pinch of salt
- Ground cinnamon and whipped cream as a garnish (optional)

Procedure

1. In a medium saucepan, whisk together the unsweetened almond milk, canned pumpkin puree, eggs, granulated sweetener, pure vanilla extract, ground cinnamon, ground nutmeg, ground ginger, ground cloves, and a pinch of salt until well combined.

2. Place the saucepan over medium heat and cook the mixture, stirring constantly, until it begins to simmer. Do not let it come to a boil.

3. Once the mixture begins to simmer, reduce the heat to low and continue to cook, stirring occasionally, for about 5-7 minutes or until slightly thickened.

4. Remove the saucepan from the heat and let the pumpkin eggnog cool to room temperature.

5. Once cooled, transfer the pumpkin eggnog to a pitcher or covered container and refrigerate it for at least 2 hours, or until well chilled.

6. Pour the pumpkin eggnog into glasses and garnish each glass with a dollop of whipped cream and a sprinkle of ground cinnamon, if desired.

Nutritional Information
- Per serving (1/4 of the recipe, without optional toppings): Calories: 60 kcal, Carbohydrates: 6g, Protein: 3g, Fat: 3g, Saturated Fat: 0.5g, Cholesterol: 95mg, Sodium: 100mg, Fiber: 2g, Sugar: 2g

Frozen Coffee Whip

Prep Time: 10 minutes
Cook Time: 0 minutes
Freezing Time: 4 hours
Servings: 2

Ingredients
- 1 cup of room temperature coffee after it has been brewed
- 1/2 cup unsweetened almond milk (or any unsweetened milk of your choice)
- 1 tablespoon unsweetened cocoa powder
- One tablespoon of raw peanut butter or almond butter
- 1 tablespoon ground flaxseeds or chia seeds (optional, for added fiber)
- 1 teaspoon pure vanilla extract
- 1-2 tablespoons granulated sweetener of your choice, such as stevia or erythritol (optional, to taste)
- Ice cubes
- Whipped cream and cocoa powder for garnish (optional)

Procedure
1. Brew 1 cup of coffee and let it cool to room temperature. Measure out the almond milk, unsweetened cocoa powder, natural almond butter or peanut butter, ground flaxseeds or chia seeds (if using), pure vanilla extract, granulated sweetener (if using), and ice cubes.

2. In a blender, add the cooled brewed coffee, almond milk, unsweetened cocoa powder, natural almond butter or peanut butter, ground flaxseeds or chia seeds (if using), pure vanilla extract, and granulated sweetener (if using).
Optional: Add a handful of ice cubes to the blender for a thicker and frostier texture.

3. Secure the lid on the blender and blend the ingredients on high speed until smooth and creamy. If needed, stop and scrape down the sides of the blender with a spatula to ensure all ingredients are fully incorporated.

4. Taste the frozen coffee whip and adjust the sweetness if necessary by adding more granulated sweetener, if desired.

5. Transfer the blended mixture into an ice cube tray and freeze for at least 4 hours, or until solid.

6. Once frozen, remove the coffee whip cubes from the ice cube tray and transfer them to a blender.
  - Blend the frozen coffee whip cubes until smooth and creamy.
  - Pour the frozen coffee whip into glasses and garnish with whipped cream and a sprinkle of cocoa powder, if desired.

Nutritional Information
- Per serving (1/2 of the recipe, without optional toppings): Calories: 70 kcal, Carbohydrates: 3g, Protein: 2g, Fat: 5g, Saturated Fat: 0.5g, Cholesterol: 0mg, Sodium: 20mg, Fiber: 2g, Sugar: 0g

Carrot and Apple Juice

Prep Time: 10 minutes
Cook Time: 0 minutes
Servings: 2

Ingredients
- 4 large carrots, washed and peeled
- 2 medium apples, washed and cored
- 1/2 inch piece of fresh ginger (optional, for added flavor)
- Ice cubes (optional, for serving)

Procedure

1. Wash and peel the carrots, then cut them into smaller pieces that will fit into your juicer chute. Wash and core the apples, then cut them into quarters or smaller pieces. If using ginger, peel it and cut it into small chunks.

2. As directed by the manufacturer, set up your juicer. Begin by juicing the carrots, followed by the apples. If using ginger, juice it along with the carrots and apples. Continue juicing until all the ingredients have been processed.

3. If you prefer a smoother juice, you can strain it through a fine mesh sieve or cheesecloth to remove any pulp. Use a spoon to press down on the pulp to extract as much liquid as possible.

4. Pour the freshly squeezed carrot and apple juice into glasses filled with ice cubes, if desired. Optionally, garnish with a slice of apple or a sprig of fresh mint for presentation.!

Nutritional Information
- Per serving (1/2 of the recipe): Calories: 80 kcal, Carbohydrates: 20g, Protein: 1g, Fat: 0g, Saturated Fat: 0g, Cholesterol: 0mg, Sodium: 60mg, Fiber: 4g, Sugar: 15g

No Sugar Raspberry Iced Tea

Prep Time: 10 minutes
Cook Time: 5 minutes
Chilling Time: 2 hours
Servings: 4

Ingredients
- 4 cups water
- 4 black tea bags (or your preferred tea variety)
- 1 cup fresh or frozen raspberries
- Juice of 1 lemon
- Ice cubes
- Fresh mint leaves for garnish (optional)

Procedure

1. Heat 4 cups of water in a medium pot until it boils. Remove the saucepan from heat and add the black tea bags. Let the tea bags steep in the hot water for 5 minutes to extract the flavor.

   - After 5 minutes, remove the tea bags from the saucepan and discard them.

2. While the tea is still warm, add the raspberries to the saucepan. Using a spoon or a masher, gently crush the raspberries to release their juices into the tea. Let the raspberry-infused tea cool to room temperature, allowing the flavors to meld together.

3. Once the tea has cooled, strain it through a fine mesh sieve or cheesecloth to remove the raspberry pulp and seeds. Using pressure, squeeze out as much liquid as you can from the raspberries.

4. Stir in the juice of 1 lemon to the strained raspberry tea. The lemon juice will add a bright, citrusy flavor to the iced tea.

5. Transfer the raspberry iced tea to a pitcher and refrigerate it for at least 2 hours, or until well chilled. Chilling the tea allows the flavors to develop and intensify.

6. Once the raspberry iced tea is chilled, fill glasses with ice cubes and pour the tea over the ice. Garnish each glass with a sprig of fresh mint leaves, if desired, for added freshness and aroma.

Nutritional Information

- Per serving (1/4 of the recipe): Calories: 5kcal, Carbohydrates: 1g, Protein: 0g, Fat: 0g, Saturated Fat: 0g, Cholesterol: 0mg, Sodium: 5mg, Fiber: 0g, Sugar: 0g

Greenland Drink

Prep Time: 5 minutes
Cook Time: 0 minutes
Servings: 2

Ingredients
- 1 cup unsweetened green tea, chilled
- 1/2 cup unsweetened coconut water
- Juice of 1 lime
- One tablespoon of maple syrup or honey (optional; adds sweetness)
- Fresh mint leaves for garnish (optional)
- Ice cubes (optional)

Procedure
1.   Brew green tea according to package instructions and let it cool to room temperature. Once cooled, chill the green tea in the refrigerator until ready to use. Measure out the unsweetened coconut water, juice of 1 lime, honey or maple syrup (if using), fresh mint leaves for garnish (if using), and ice cubes (if desired).

2. In a pitcher or large glass, combine the chilled green tea, unsweetened coconut water, and juice of 1 lime. Stir well to combine.
 Optional: If you prefer a sweeter drink, you can add a tablespoon of honey or maple syrup to the mixture and stir until dissolved.

3. Pour the Drink into glasses filled with ice cubes, if desired.
   - Garnish each glass with fresh mint leaves for added freshness and aroma, if using.
   - Serve immediately and enjoy this refreshing and hydrating beverage!

Nutritional Information
- Per serving (1/2 of the recipe): Calories: 20 kcal, Carbohydrates: 5g, Protein: 0g, Fat: 0g, Saturated Fat: 0g, Cholesterol: 0mg, Sodium: 25mg, Fiber: 0g, Sugar: 3g

Berry Delicious Nutty Milkshake

Prep Time: 5 minutes
Cook Time: 0 minutes
Servings: 2

Ingredients
- 1 cup unsweetened almond milk (or any unsweetened milk of your choice)
- 1 cup mixed berries (such as strawberries, blueberries, and raspberries), fresh or frozen
- 2 tablespoons unsalted mixed nuts (such as almonds, walnuts, and pecans)
- 1 tablespoon ground flaxseeds or chia seeds
- 1 tablespoon natural almond butter or peanut butter (unsweetened)
- 1/2 teaspoon pure vanilla extract
- Ice cubes (optional, for a thicker texture)
- Pinch of cinnamon (optional)
- Fresh berries and chopped nuts for garnish (optional)

Procedure
1. Measure out the unsweetened almond milk, mixed berries, unsalted mixed nuts, ground flaxseeds or chia seeds, natural almond butter or peanut butter, and pure vanilla extract.

2. In a blender, add the unsweetened almond milk, mixed berries, unsalted mixed nuts, ground flaxseeds or chia seeds, natural almond butter or peanut butter, and pure vanilla extract.
   Optional: For added flavor, add a pinch of cinnamon. If you prefer a thicker milkshake, you can add a handful of ice cubes to the blender.

3. Secure the lid on the blender and blend the ingredients on high speed until smooth and creamy. If needed, stop and scrape down the sides of the blender with a spatula to ensure all ingredients are fully incorporated.

4. Taste the milkshake and adjust the sweetness or thickness if necessary. If you prefer a sweeter milkshake, you can add a teaspoon of honey or maple syrup, although the natural sweetness of the berries should suffice for most palates.

5. Pour the Milkshake into glasses and garnish with fresh berries and chopped nuts, if desired.

Nutritional Information
-Per serving (1/2 of the recipe): Calories: 180 kcal, Carbohydrates: 14g, Protein: 6g, Fat: 12g, Saturated Fat: 1.5g, Cholesterol: 0mg, Sodium: 80mg, Fiber: 6g, Sugar: 6g

Peanut Butter Oatmeal Smoothie

Prep Time: 5 minutes
Cook Time: 0 minutes
Servings: 2

Ingredients
- 1 ripe banana, peeled and sliced
- 1/4 cup rolled oats (use gluten-free oats if needed)
- 2 tablespoons natural peanut butter (unsweetened)
- 1 cup unsweetened almond milk (or any unsweetened milk of your choice)
- 1 tablespoon ground flaxseeds or chia seeds
- 1/2 teaspoon pure vanilla extract
- Ice cubes (optional, for a thicker texture)
- Pinch of cinnamon (optional, for added flavor)

Procedure
1. Peel and slice the ripe banana. Measure out the rolled oats, natural peanut butter, ground flaxseeds or chia seeds, and unsweetened almond milk.

2. In a blender, add the sliced banana, rolled oats, natural peanut butter, ground flaxseeds or chia seeds, unsweetened almond milk, and pure vanilla extract.
  Optional: Add a pinch of cinnamon for added flavor. If you prefer a thicker smoothie, you can add a handful of ice cubes to the blender.

3. Secure the lid on the blender and blend the ingredients on high speed until smooth and creamy. If needed, stop and scrape down the sides of the blender with a spatula to ensure all ingredients are fully incorporated.

4. Taste the smoothie and adjust the sweetness or thickness if necessary. If you prefer a sweeter smoothie, you can add a teaspoon of honey or maple syrup, although the natural sweetness of the banana should suffice for most palates.

Nutritional Information
- Per serving (1/2 of the recipe): Calories: 280 kcal, Carbohydrates: 31g, Protein: 9g,
Fat: 15g, Saturated Fat: 2.5g, Cholesterol: 0mg, Sodium: 110mg, Fiber: 6g, Sugar: 10g

Strawberry Pineapple Smoothie

Prep Time: 5 minutes
Cook Time: 0 minutes
Servings: 2

Ingredients
- 1 cup frozen strawberries
- 1 cup frozen pineapple chunks
- 1 cup unsweetened almond milk (or any unsweetened milk of your choice)
- 1/2 cup plain Greek yogurt (unsweetened)
- 1 tablespoon ground flaxseeds (optional, for added fiber and omega-3 fatty acids)
- 1 teaspoon honey or maple syrup (optional, for added sweetness)
- Ice cubes (optional, for a thicker texture)

Procedure
1. If using fresh strawberries and pineapple, wash and chop them into small pieces.
Alternatively, you can use pre-packaged frozen strawberries and pineapple chunks for
convenience.

2. In a blender, add the frozen strawberries, frozen pineapple chunks, unsweetened
almond milk, plain Greek yogurt, ground flaxseeds (if using), and honey or maple
syrup (if using).
Optional: If you prefer a thicker smoothie, you can add a few ice cubes to the blender.

3. Secure the lid on the blender and blend the ingredients on high speed until smooth
and creamy. If needed, stop and scrape down the sides of the blender with a spatula to
ensure all ingredients are fully incorporated.

4. Taste the smoothie and adjust the sweetness if necessary by adding more honey or maple syrup, if desired. Keep in mind that the natural sweetness of the strawberries and pineapple may be sufficient for your taste preferences.

5. Pour the smoothie into glasses and garnish with a slice of strawberry or pineapple, if desired.

Nutritional Information
-Per serving (1/2 of the recipe): Calories: 140 kcal, Carbohydrates: 25g, Protein: 7g, Fat: 2.5g, Saturated Fat: 0g, Cholesterol: 0mg, Sodium: 90mg, Fiber: 5g, Sugar: 16g

LUNCH RECIPES

Whole-Grain Pasta With Lean Protein and Veggies

Prep Time: 15 minutes
Cook Time: 15 minutes
Servings: 4

Ingredients
- 8 ounces whole-grain pasta (such as whole wheat or brown rice pasta)
- 1 tablespoon olive oil
- 1 small onion, diced
- 2 cloves garlic, minced
- 2 cups chopped mixed vegetables (such as bell peppers, zucchini, broccoli, and carrots)
- 8 ounces lean protein (such as skinless chicken breast, turkey breast, or tofu), diced or sliced
- 1 cup low-sodium chicken or vegetable broth
- 1 teaspoon dried Italian herbs (such as basil, oregano, and thyme)
- Salt and pepper to taste
- Grated Parmesan cheese for serving (optional)
- Parsley or fresh parsley for garnish (optional)

Procedure

1. Heat a big saucepan of salted water till it boils. When the water boils, add the whole-grain pasta and cook it until al dente, following the directions on the package. After the pasta has cooked, drain it and set it aside.

2. In a large skillet over medium heat, warm the olive oil while the pasta cooks. Add the diced onion and minced garlic to the skillet and sauté for 2-3 minutes, or until fragrant and translucent. Add the chopped mixed vegetables to the skillet and cook for 5-7 minutes, or until they are tender-crisp.

3. Push the vegetables to one side of the skillet and add the diced or sliced lean protein to the other side. Cook the protein for 4-5 minutes, or until it is cooked through.

4. Once the vegetables and protein are cooked, add the cooked pasta to the skillet. Pour the low-sodium chicken or vegetable broth over the pasta, vegetables, and protein. Sprinkle the dried Italian herbs over the mixture.

5. Season with salt and pepper to taste. Stir everything together until well and heated through.

6. Divide among serving plates or bowls. Sprinkle grated Parmesan cheese over each serving, if desired. Garnish with fresh basil or parsley leaves for added flavor and freshness.

Notes
• Enhance the flavor of the dish by adding ingredients such as sun-dried tomatoes, olives, capers, or roasted garlic. These flavorful additions can elevate the taste of the pasta dish and add variety to the meal.

• You can also use plant-based protein options like tempeh or seitan for a vegetarian or vegan version of the dish.

• Increase the nutritional value of the pasta dish by adding leafy greens such as spinach, kale, or Swiss chard. Simply wilt the greens in the skillet along with the other vegetables for added vitamins and minerals.

• While whole-grain pasta is a nutritious choice, you can also opt for other types of pasta such as lentil or chickpea pasta for added protein and fiber. These alternative pasta options are gluten-free and suitable for individuals with gluten sensitivities or allergies.

• If you prefer a dairy-free option, you can omit the Parmesan cheese or use a dairy-free alternative such as nutritional yeast or dairy-free cheese. This allows individuals with lactose intolerance or dairy allergies to enjoy the dish without any issues.

Nutritional Information (per serving)
- Calories: 350 kcal
- Protein: 25g
- Fat: 8g

- Carbohydrates: 45g
- Fiber: 7g
- Sugars: 5g

Low-Sodium Bean Soup With a Cheese Stick and Sunflower Seeds

Prep Time: 10 minutes
Cook Time: 30 minutes
Servings: 4

Ingredients
- 1 tablespoon olive oil
- 1 small onion, diced
- 2 cloves garlic, minced
- 2 carrots, diced
- 2 celery stalks, diced
- 1 teaspoon dried thyme
- 1 teaspoon dried oregano
- 1/2 teaspoon smoked paprika
- 4 cups low-sodium vegetable broth
- 2 cans (15 ounces each) low-sodium beans (such as black beans, kidney beans, or cannellini beans), drained and rinsed
- Salt and pepper to taste
- 4 cheese sticks (such as mozzarella or cheddar)
- 1/4 cup unsalted sunflower seeds

Procedure
1. Heat the olive oil in a large pot over medium heat. Add the diced onion and minced garlic to the pot and sauté for 2-3 minutes, or until fragrant and translucent.

2. Add the diced carrots and celery to the pot with the onions and garlic. Sprinkle the dried thyme, dried oregano, and smoked paprika over the vegetables. Stir to coat the vegetables evenly with the spices.

3. Pour the low-sodium vegetable broth into the pot with the vegetables and spices. Bring the soup to a simmer and cook for 15-20 minutes, or until the vegetables are tender.

4. Once the vegetables are tender, add the drained and rinsed low-sodium beans to the pot. Stir to combine and continue to simmer the soup for an additional 5-10 minutes to allow the flavors to meld together.

5. Season the soup with salt and pepper to taste, keeping in mind that the vegetable broth and beans are already low in sodium.

6. Divide the Low-Sodium Bean Soup among serving bowls. Serve each bowl of soup with a cheese stick and a sprinkle of unsalted sunflower seeds on top for added flavor and texture.

Notes
• Boost the nutritional content of the soup by adding additional vegetables such as diced bell peppers, diced tomatoes, or chopped spinach. These vegetables not only add color and flavor but also provide extra vitamins and minerals.

• Feel free to use any variety of low-sodium beans in the soup, depending on your preferences. You can mix and match beans such as black beans, kidney beans, cannellini beans, or chickpeas for added variety and texture.

• If you prefer a creamier soup, you can blend a portion of the soup using an immersion blender or traditional blender until smooth. Then, stir the blended soup back into the pot for a creamy texture without adding cream or dairy.

• Pair the Low-Sodium Bean Soup with a slice of whole grain bread or a whole grain roll for a complete and satisfying meal. The additional fiber from the whole grains will help keep you feeling full and satisfied.

Nutritional Information (per serving)
- Calories: 350 kcal
- Protein: 17g
- Fat: 17g
- Carbohydrates: 38g
- Fiber: 10g
- Sugars: 5g

Turkey & Cheddar Lettuce Wraps

Prep Time: 15 minutes
Cook Time 10 minutes
Servings: 4

Ingredients
- 1 pound lean ground turkey
- 1 tablespoon olive oil
- 1 small onion, diced
- 2 cloves garlic, minced
- 1 teaspoon ground cumin
- 1 teaspoon chili powder
- 1/2 teaspoon paprika
- Salt and pepper to taste
- Eight huge lettuce leaves, romaine or iceberg
- 1 cup shredded cheddar cheese
- 1 tomato, diced
- 1/2 avocado, sliced
- 1/4 cup salsa (optional)
- Fresh cilantro leaves for garnish (optional)

Procedure
1. In a large saucepan, warm up olive oil over medium heat. Add the diced onion and minced garlic to the skillet and sauté for 2-3 minutes, or until fragrant and translucent. Add the lean ground turkey to the skillet and cook, breaking it apart with a spoon, until browned and cooked through, about 5-7 minutes.

2. Stir in the ground cumin, chili powder, paprika, salt, and pepper, and cook for an additional 2-3 minutes to allow the flavors to meld together.

3. Arrange the large lettuce leaves on a clean work surface. Spoon the cooked turkey mixture onto each lettuce leaf, dividing it evenly among them. Top each lettuce wrap

with shredded cheddar cheese, diced tomato, sliced avocado, and a dollop of salsa, if desired.

4. Carefully roll up each lettuce leaf to enclose the filling, like a burrito or wrap. Secure the wraps with toothpicks if necessary to hold them together.

5. Arrange the Turkey & Cheddar Lettuce Wraps on a serving platter. If desired,Garnish with fresh cilantro leaves.

Notes
• Feel free to customize the filling ingredients based on your preferences and dietary restrictions. You can add or omit ingredients such as diced bell peppers, black beans, corn kernels, or jalapeños to suit your taste. This allows you to create a variety of flavor combinations and tailor the wraps to your liking.

• For extra flavor and moisture, consider adding a dollop of Greek yogurt, sour cream, or guacamole to each lettuce wrap before rolling them up. These creamy sauces add richness and texture to the wraps and complement the savory turkey and cheddar filling.

• If you enjoy spicy food, you can add a sprinkle of crushed red pepper flakes or a dash of hot sauce to the turkey mixture for a kick of heat. Alternatively, you can include diced jalapeños or serrano peppers for an extra spicy kick.

• Enhance the texture of the wraps by adding crunchy toppings such as sliced radishes, shredded carrots, or crushed tortilla chips. These toppings add a satisfying crunch to each bite and provide additional flavor and nutrients to the wraps.

• Serve with a side of salsa, ranch dressing, or barbecue sauce for dipping. These sauces add extra flavor and moisture to the wraps and can be used as a dipping sauce or drizzled over the top for added flavor.

• Experiment with different types of lettuce leaves for the wraps, such as butter lettuce, green leaf lettuce, or Bibb lettuce. Each variety offers a unique texture and flavor profile, allowing you to create a diverse range of wraps to suit your preferences.

Nutritional Information (per serving)
- Calories: 320 kcal
- Protein: 25g
- Fat: 18g

- Carbohydrates: 15g
- Fiber: 6g
- Sugars: 4g

Keto Sushi

Prep Time: 20 minutes
Cook Time: 0 minutes
Servings: 2-3

Ingredients
- 1 large cucumber
- 4 oz cream cheese, softened
- 4 ounces of cooked shrimp or smoked salmon
- 1 avocado, sliced
- 2 tablespoons soy sauce or tamari (for dipping, optional)
- Ginger pickles with wasabi paste (optional for serving)

Procedure
1. After cleaning, trim the ends of the cucumber. Thinly slice the cucumber lengthwise into long, thin strips using a mandoline slicer or vegetable peeler.. Lay the cucumber strips flat on a clean kitchen towel and gently pat them dry to remove excess moisture.

2. Lay one cucumber strip flat on a cutting board. Spread a thin layer of softened cream cheese evenly over the entire surface of the cucumber strip. Place a thin layer of smoked salmon or cooked shrimp along one edge of the cucumber strip.

3. Place a few slices of avocado on top of the salmon or shrimp. Carefully roll up the cucumber strip, starting from the edge with the filling, to form a sushi roll. Repeat this process with the remaining cucumber strips and filling ingredients.

4. Use a sharp knife to slice each sushi roll into bite-sized pieces, about 1 inch thick. Arrange the Keto Sushi rolls on a serving platter. Serve with soy sauce or tamari for dipping, if desired, and garnish with wasabi paste and pickled ginger for added flavor.

<u>**Notes**</u>

• Enhance the texture and flavor of the sushi rolls by adding crunchy vegetables such as sliced bell peppers, shredded carrots, or cucumber matchsticks along with the avocado filling. These vegetables add freshness and crunch to the rolls, making them even more satisfying to eat.

• Get creative with the fillings for the Keto Sushi rolls by using different proteins and flavor combinations. You can try filling the rolls with cooked crab meat, tuna salad, or grilled chicken for variety. You can also add sliced jalapeños or cream cheese for a spicy kick.

• Instead of traditional soy sauce or tamari, consider serving the Keto Sushi rolls with alternative dipping sauces that are low in carbohydrates and sugar. Options include coconut aminos, sesame oil, or a homemade dipping sauce made with vinegar, ginger, and garlic.

• If you prefer a more traditional sushi experience, you can wrap the cucumber "rice" and fill ingredients in sheets of nori (seaweed) before rolling them up. Nori sheets add a savory flavor and authentic sushi texture to the rolls, making them even more satisfying.

• Before serving, sprinkle the Keto Sushi rolls with toasted sesame seeds for added flavor and visual appeal. Sesame seeds add a nutty taste and crunchy texture to the rolls, enhancing their overall presentation.

• Pair with low-carb side dishes such as seaweed salad, cauliflower rice, or a mixed green salad with ginger dressing. These side dishes complement the sushi rolls and provide additional nutrients and flavor to the meal.

Nutritional Information (per serving, based on 3 servings)
- Calories: 320 kcal
- Protein: 12g
- Fat: 26g
- Carbohydrates: 9g
- Fiber: 5g
- Sugars: 2g

Stuffed Potato with Salsa and Beans

Prep Time: 15 minutes
Cook Time: 45 minutes
Servings: 4

Ingredients
- 4 medium-sized russet potatoes
- 1 tablespoon olive oil
- 1 small onion, diced
- 2 cloves garlic, minced
- 1 bell pepper, diced (any color)
- One can (15 ounces) of black beans rinsed and drained.
- 1 cup salsa (homemade or store-bought)
- 1 teaspoon ground cumin
- 1 teaspoon chili powder
- Salt and pepper to taste

Optional toppings: shredded cheddar cheese, diced avocado, chopped cilantro, Greek yogurt or sour cream

Procedure

1. Preheat your oven to 400°F (200°C). Scrub the russet potatoes clean under running water and pat them dry with a kitchen towel. To release steam while baking, pierce each potato multiple times using a fork. Arrange the potatoes on a baking pan covered with aluminum foil or parchment paper.

2. Place the baking sheet with the potatoes in the preheated oven and bake for 45-60 minutes, or until the potatoes are tender when pierced with a fork. The cooking time may vary depending on the size and thickness of the potatoes.

3. While the potatoes are baking, heat the olive oil in a large skillet over medium heat. Add the diced onion and minced garlic to the skillet and sauté for 2-3 minutes, or until fragrant and translucent.

4. Add the diced bell pepper to the skillet with the onions and garlic, and cook for an additional 2-3 minutes, or until the pepper begins to soften. Then, add the drained and rinsed black beans to the skillet, along with the ground cumin, chili powder, salt, and pepper. Stir to combine and cook for another 2-3 minutes to allow the flavors to meld together.

5. Pour the salsa into the skillet with the bean mixture and stir to combine. Cook for an additional 2-3 minutes, or until the salsa is heated through and the flavors have blended together.

6. Once the potatoes are cooked, remove them from the oven and let them cool slightly. Using a sharp knife, make a slit lengthwise down the center of each potato, being careful not to cut all the way through. Gently press the ends of each potato to open them up slightly.

7. Spoon the salsa and bean mixture generously into each potato, filling the center cavity. Top each stuffed potato with optional toppings such as shredded cheddar cheese, diced avocado, chopped cilantro, or a dollop of Greek yogurt or sour cream.

Nutritional Information (per serving)
- Calories: 300 kcal
- Protein: 10g
- Fat: 5g
- Carbohydrates: 55g
- Fiber: 10g
- Sugars: 5g

Lean Pork and Veggie Tacos or Quesadillas

Prep Time: 15 minutes
Cook Time: 20 minutes
Servings: 4

<u>For the Pork</u>:

- 1 pound lean pork tenderloin, thinly sliced
- 1 tablespoon olive oil
- 1 teaspoon ground cumin
- 1 teaspoon chili powder
- 1/2 teaspoon paprika

For the Veggie Filling:
- 1 tablespoon olive oil
- 1 small onion, diced
- 1 bell pepper, diced (any color)
- 1 zucchini, diced
- 1 cup sliced mushrooms
- 2 cloves garlic, minced
- Salt and pepper to taste

For Serving:
- Eight tiny corn or whole wheat tortillas
Optional toppings: shredded lettuce, diced tomatoes, sliced avocado, Greek yogurt or sour cream, salsa

Procedure

1. In a small bowl, combine the ground cumin, chili powder, paprika, salt, and pepper. Rub the spice mixture evenly over the thinly sliced pork tenderloin.

2. Heat the olive oil in a large skillet over medium-high heat. Add the seasoned pork slices to the skillet and cook for 3-4 minutes per side, or until browned and cooked through. Remove from heat and set aside.

3. In the same skillet, heat another tablespoon of olive oil over medium heat. Add the diced onion, bell pepper, zucchini, mushrooms, and minced garlic to the skillet. Season with salt and pepper to taste. Cook the vegetables for 5-7 minutes, or until they are tender and lightly browned.

4. **For Tacos**: Warm the tortillas in a dry skillet or microwave. Divide the cooked pork slices and veggie filling evenly among the tortillas. Add optional toppings such as shredded lettuce, diced tomatoes, sliced avocado, Greek yogurt or sour cream, and salsa.

For Quesadillas: Place 4 tortillas on a clean work surface. Divide the cooked pork slices and veggie filling evenly among the tortillas. Top each with another tortilla to create a sandwich.

5. Heat a non-stick skillet over medium heat. Place one quesadilla in the skillet and cook for 2-3 minutes per side, or until golden brown and crispy. Repeat with the remaining quesadillas. Serve

<u>**Notes**</u>
• Experiment with different seasonings and herbs to add extra flavor to the pork and veggie filling. You can try adding ingredients like smoked paprika, oregano, garlic powder, or a squeeze of fresh lime juice for added zest.

• Boost the nutritional value of the tacos or quesadillas by incorporating healthy fats. Consider adding sliced avocado or a drizzle of olive oil to provide heart-healthy monounsaturated fats that help promote satiety and provide essential nutrients.

• Opt for whole wheat tortillas instead of traditional white flour tortillas to increase the fiber content and improve blood sugar control. Whole wheat tortillas are higher in fiber and nutrients, making them a healthier choice for individuals with type 2 diabetes.

• For a meatless option, you can omit the pork and increase the amount of veggies in the filling. Consider adding additional vegetables such as diced tomatoes, corn kernels, or black beans for added texture and protein.

• Pair the tacos or quesadillas with homemade fresh salsa for added flavor and freshness. You can make a simple salsa using diced tomatoes, onions, cilantro, jalapeños, lime juice, and a pinch of salt. Fresh salsa adds a burst of flavor and nutrients without added sugars or preservatives.

• For a spicy kick, add chopped jalapeños or a sprinkle of crushed red pepper flakes to the veggie filling. Spicy ingredients not only add flavor but also help rev up metabolism and improve blood circulation.

Nutritional Information (per serving, based on 2 tacos or 1 quesadilla)
- Calories: 350 kcal (tacos), 400 kcal (quesadilla)
- Protein: 25g
- Fat: 10g

- Carbohydrates: 40g (tacos), 30g (quesadilla)
- Fiber: 8g
- Sugars: 5g

Sweet Potato Bowl with Black Beans and Quinoa Tofu Stir-Fry

Prep Time: 15 minutes
Cook Time: 45 minutes
Servings: 4

For the Sweet Potato Bowl

- 2 large sweet potatoes, peeled and cubed
- 1 tablespoon olive oil
- 1 teaspoon smoked paprika
- 1 teaspoon garlic powder
- Salt and pepper to taste
- One can (15 ounces) black beans, rinsed and drained

Optional toppings: diced avocado, sliced green onions, Greek yogurt or sour cream

For the Quinoa Tofu Stir-Fry:

- 1 cup quinoa, rinsed
- 2 cups vegetable broth or water
- 1 tablespoon sesame oil
- 1 block (14 ounces) extra-firm tofu, pressed and cubed
- 2 cups mixed vegetables (such as bell peppers, broccoli, carrots, snap peas)
- 2 cloves garlic, minced
- 2 tablespoons soy sauce or tamari
- 1 tablespoon rice vinegar
- 1 tablespoon maple syrup or honey (optional)
- Sesame seeds for garnish (optional)

Procedure

1. Preheat your oven to 400°F (200°C). In a large bowl, toss the cubed sweet potatoes with olive oil, smoked paprika, garlic powder, salt, and pepper until evenly coated. Spread the seasoned sweet potatoes in a single layer on a baking sheet lined with parchment paper or aluminum foil.

2. Roast the sweet potatoes in the preheated oven for 25-30 minutes, or until tender and lightly browned, stirring halfway through the cooking time.

3. In a medium saucepan, bring the vegetable broth or water to a boil. Add the rinsed quinoa to the boiling broth, reduce the heat to low, cover, and simmer for 15-20 minutes, or until the quinoa is cooked and the liquid is absorbed. Fluff the quinoa with a fork and set aside.

3. Heat the sesame oil in a large skillet or wok over medium-high heat. Add the cubed tofu to the skillet and cook for 5-7 minutes, or until golden brown and crispy on all sides. Remove the tofu from the skillet and set aside. In the same skillet, add the mixed vegetables and minced garlic. Stir-fry for 3-4 minutes, or until the vegetables are tender-crisp.

4. Return the cooked tofu to the skillet. Add the soy sauce or tamari, rice vinegar, and maple syrup or honey (if using). Stir to coat the tofu and vegetables evenly with the sauce. Cook for an additional 2-3 minutes, or until heated through.

5. Divide the roasted sweet potatoes, cooked quinoa, black beans, and tofu stir-fry among serving bowls. Top each bowl with optional toppings such as diced avocado, sliced green onions, and a dollop of Greek yogurt or sour cream. Garnish with sesame seeds if desired.

Nutritional Information (per serving)
- Calories: 400 kcal
- Protein: 18g
- Fat: 12g
- Carbohydrates: 60g
- Fiber: 14g
- Sugars: 7g

Salmon Salad with White Beans

Prep Time: 15 minutes
Cook Time: 15 minutes
Servings: 4

For the Salmon
- 4 salmon filets, each weighing around 4 ounces
- 1 tablespoon olive oil
- 1 teaspoon lemon zest
- 1 teaspoon dried dill
- Salt and pepper to taste

For the Salad:
- One can (15 ounces) of white beans, rinsed and drained
- 4 cups mixed salad greens
- 1 cup cherry tomatoes, halved
- 1/2 cucumber, sliced
- 1/4 red onion, thinly sliced
- **Optional toppings**: sliced avocado, crumbled feta cheese, sliced olives

For the Dressing:
- 2 tablespoons olive oil
- 1 tablespoon lemon juice
- 1 teaspoon Dijon mustard
- 1 clove garlic, minced
- Salt and pepper to taste

Procedure
1. Preheat your oven to 400°F (200°C). Arrange the salmon filets onto a baking sheet that has been covered with aluminum foil or parchment paper. In a small bowl, mix together the olive oil, lemon zest, dried dill, salt, and pepper. Brush the seasoned olive oil mixture over the salmon filets.

2. Bake the salmon in the preheated oven for 12-15 minutes, or until the salmon is cooked through and flakes easily with a fork.

3. In a large mixing bowl, combine the drained and rinsed white beans, mixed salad greens, cherry tomatoes, sliced cucumber, and thinly sliced red onion. Mix the salad ingredients until well distributed

4.   In a small bowl, whisk together the olive oil, lemon juice, Dijon mustard, minced garlic, salt, and pepper until well combined. Divide the prepared salad mixture among serving plates or bowls.

5. Place a baked salmon filet on top of each salad portion. Drizzle the prepared dressing over the salads. Garnish with optional toppings such as sliced avocado, crumbled feta cheese, or sliced olives.

Nutritional Information (per serving)
- Calories: 350 kcal
- Protein: 25g
- Fat: 18g
- Carbohydrates: 20g
- Fiber: 6g
- Sugars: 3g

DINNER RECIPES

Grilled Chicken with Farro & Roasted Cauliflower

Prep Time: 15 minutes
Cook Time: 35 minutes
Servings: 4

Ingredients
- 4 boneless, skinless chicken breasts
- 1 cup farro
- 1 head cauliflower, cut into florets
- 2 tablespoons olive oil, divided
- 2 cloves garlic, minced
- 1 teaspoon dried thyme
- 1 teaspoon paprika
- Salt and pepper to taste
- Fresh parsley for garnish

Procedure

1. Preheat your grill to medium-high heat. Preheat a gas grill by turning on all of the burners. In the event that you're using a charcoal barbecue, light the charcoal and allow it to burn until gray ash covers the coals.

2. Drizzle some olive oil and season the chicken breasts with salt and pepper. To provide an even coating, rub the seasonings into the chicken.

3. Place the seasoned chicken breasts on the preheated grill. Cook for 6-8 minutes per side, or until the chicken is cooked through and reaches an internal temperature of 165°F (75°C). Depending on the thickness of the chicken breasts, different cooking

periods may apply. After cooking, take the chicken from the grill and give it some time to rest before slicing.

4. While the chicken is grilling, rinse the farro under cold water. In a medium saucepan, bring 2 cups of water to a boil. Add the rinsed farro and reduce the heat to low. Cover and simmer for 20-25 minutes, or until the farro is tender and has absorbed the water. After cooking, take it off the heat and cover it for five minutes before fluffing with a fork.

5. While the chicken and farro are cooking, preheat your oven to 400°F (200°C). In a large mixing bowl, toss the cauliflower florets with 1 tablespoon of olive oil, minced garlic, dried thyme, paprika, salt, and pepper until evenly coated. Spread the seasoned cauliflower in a single layer on a baking sheet lined with parchment paper. Roast in the preheated oven for 20-25 minutes, or until the cauliflower is tender and golden brown, stirring halfway through cooking.

6. To serve, divide the cooked farro among serving plates. Top with sliced grilled chicken breasts and roasted cauliflower florets. Garnish with freshly chopped parsley for a pop of color and flavor.

Nutritional Information
Calories: 420 kcal,
Carbohydrates: 34g
Protein: 36g
Fat: 15g,
Saturated Fat: 2.5g
Cholesterol: 90mg,
Sodium: 160mg
Fiber: 7g,
Sugar: 4g

Kale, Sausage & Pepper Pasta

Prep Time: 15 minutes
Cook Time: 25 minutes
Servings: 4

Ingredients

- 8 ounces whole wheat or whole grain pasta
- 4 links of Italian turkey or chicken sausage, sliced
- 1 tablespoon olive oil
- 2 cloves garlic, minced
- 1 red bell pepper, thinly sliced
- 1 yellow bell pepper, thinly sliced
- one bunch of chopped, bite-sized kale leaves
- 1/4 teaspoon red pepper flakes (optional)
- Salt and pepper to taste
- Grated Parmesan cheese for garnish (optional)

Procedure

1. Bring a large pot of salted water to a boil, add the pasta, and cook it as directed on the package until it's al dente. Drain the cooked pasta, reserving 1/2 cup of pasta water, and set aside.

2. In a large skillet over medium heat, warm the olive oil while the pasta cooks. Add the sliced sausage links to the skillet and cook until browned on both sides, about 5-7 minutes. After removing it from the skillet, set aside the browned sausage.

3. In the same skillet, add the minced garlic and sliced bell peppers. Sauté for 2-3 minutes, or until the peppers start to soften. Add the torn kale leaves to the skillet, along with the red pepper flakes (if using). Cook for an additional 3-4 minutes, stirring occasionally, until the kale is wilted and tender.

4. Return the cooked sausage to the skillet with the sautéed vegetables. Add the cooked pasta to the skillet, along with the reserved pasta water. To combine all the ingredients and heat through, stir well. Season with salt and pepper to taste.

5. Divide among serving plates. Garnish with grated Parmesan cheese, if desired, for extra flavor. Serve hot and enjoy!

<u>Notes</u>

• You can use any type of sausage you prefer, such as pork, beef, or plant-based sausage. Additionally, you can adjust the amount of garlic, red pepper flakes, and Parmesan cheese according to your taste preferences.

• When preparing the kale, be sure to remove the tough stems and tear the leaves into bite-sized pieces. Massaging the kale with a bit of olive oil and lemon juice before cooking can help soften its texture and reduce bitterness.

• It pairs well with a side salad or steamed vegetables for added nutrients and fiber. You can also serve it with a slice of whole grain bread or garlic bread for a complete and satisfying meal.

• This pasta dish makes excellent leftovers and can be stored in an airtight container in the refrigerator for up to 3-4 days. Simply reheat individual portions in the microwave or on the stovetop with a splash of water to prevent drying out.

Nutritional Information
Calories: 380 kcal
Carbohydrates: 45g
Protein: 22g
Fat: 14g
Saturated Fat: 3g
Cholesterol: 50mg,
Sodium: 550mg
Fiber: 6g
Sugar: 4g

Hamburger Steak with Onions and Gravy

Prep Time: 15 minutes
Cook Time: 25 minutes
Servings: 4

Ingredients
- 1 pound lean ground beef (at least 90% lean)
- 1/4 cup whole wheat or gluten-free breadcrumbs
- 1/4 cup finely chopped onion

- 1 teaspoon garlic powder
- 1 teaspoon Worcestershire sauce
- 2 large onions, thinly sliced
- 2 tablespoons olive oil
- 2 tablespoons all-purpose flour (or cornstarch for a gluten-free option)
- 2 cups low-sodium beef broth
- 1 teaspoon Worcestershire sauce
- Salt and pepper to taste
- Chopped fresh parsley for garnish (optional)

Procedure

1. In a large mixing bowl, combine the lean ground beef, breadcrumbs, finely chopped onion, garlic powder, Worcestershire sauce, salt, and pepper. Use your hands to mix the ingredients until well combined. Divide the mixture into four equal portions and shape them into oval-shaped patties, about 1/2 inch thick. Set aside.

2. In a large saucepan, warm up olive oil on medium heat. Add the thinly sliced onions to the skillet and cook, stirring occasionally, for 10-12 minutes, or until the onions are caramelized and golden brown. After taking the onions out of the skillet, set them aside.

3. Place the hamburger steaks in the same skillet. Cook until browned and well cooked, 4–5 minutes per side. Remove the cooked hamburger steaks from the skillet and set aside.

4. In the same skillet, add the all-purpose flour (or cornstarch) to the remaining drippings from the hamburger steaks. Cook, stirring constantly, for 1-2 minutes to cook off the raw flour taste. Gradually whisk in the low-sodium beef broth and Worcestershire sauce until smooth. Bring the mixture to a simmer and cook for 3-4 minutes, or until the gravy has thickened to your desired consistency. Add salt and pepper to taste when preparing the gravy.

5. Return the cooked hamburger steaks and caramelized onions to the skillet with the gravy. Spoon some of the gravy over the hamburger steaks and onions.
    - Cook for an additional 2-3 minutes, or until the hamburger steaks are heated through and the flavors have melded together.

<u>Notes</u>

• If the gravy is not thick enough to your liking, you can create a slurry by mixing 1-2 tablespoons of cornstarch with equal parts water until smooth. Gradually stir the slurry into the simmering gravy until it reaches the desired thickness.

• Feel free to customize the seasoning of the hamburger steaks and gravy according to your taste preferences. You can add herbs such as thyme or rosemary to the hamburger steak mixture for extra flavor. Similarly, you can add a splash of red wine or balsamic vinegar to the gravy for depth of flavor.

• For added texture and flavor, consider adding sliced mushrooms to the onions while caramelizing them. Mushrooms pair well with the savory flavors of the hamburger steaks and gravy, adding an earthy richness to the dish.

• If you're watching your sodium intake, opt for low-sodium beef broth and Worcestershire sauce in the recipe. You can also reduce the amount of salt added to the hamburger steak mixture and gravy to control the overall sodium content of the dish.

• You can prepare the hamburger steaks and caramelized onions in advance and store them in the refrigerator for up to 24 hours before cooking. Simply reheat them in the skillet with the gravy when ready to serve for a quick and convenient meal.

• Serve with your favorite side dishes such as mashed potatoes, steamed rice, or roasted vegetables. For a lower-carb option, serve the dish with cauliflower mash or cauliflower rice

Nutritional Information
Calories: 350 kcal
Carbohydrates: 15g
Protein: 25g
Fat: 20g
Saturated Fat: 6g
Cholesterol: 70mg
Sodium: 450mg
Fiber: 2g
Sugar: 3g

Chicken Meatballs With Whipped Tahini and Arugula

Prep Time: 20 minutes
Cook Time: 20 minutes
Servings: 4

Ingredients
- 1 pound ground chicken
- 1/4 cup whole wheat or gluten free breadcrumbs
- 1/4 cup grated Parmesan cheese
- 1 egg
- 2 cloves garlic, minced
- 1 teaspoon dried oregano
- 1 teaspoon dried basil
- 2 tablespoons olive oil
- ¼ pepper
- 1/4 cup tahini
- 2 tablespoons lemon juice
- 2 tablespoons water
- 1 clove garlic, minced
- Salt to taste
- 4 cups baby arugula
- 1 tablespoon olive oil
- 1 tablespoon lemon juice
- Salt and pepper to taste

Procedure

1. In a large mixing bowl, combine ground chicken, breadcrumbs, grated Parmesan cheese, egg, minced garlic, dried oregano, dried basil, salt, and pepper. Mix the ingredients with your hand until well combined.

   - Form the mixture into golf ball-sized meatballs, rolling them gently between your palms. The formed meatballs should be placed on a baking sheet or platter.

2. In a big skillet over medium heat, warm up the olive oil. Once the oil is hot, add the meatballs to the skillet, making sure not to overcrowd the pan. Cook the meatballs in batches if necessary. Cook the meatballs for 10-12 minutes, turning occasionally, until

they are golden brown and cooked through. The internal temperature should reach 165°F (75°C).

After cooking, move the meatballs to a plate covered with paper towels so that any extra oil may be drained off

3. In a small bowl, whisk together tahini, lemon juice, water, minced garlic, and a pinch of salt until smooth and creamy. If the mixture is too thick, you can add more water until you reach your desired consistency. Set aside.

4. In a large mixing bowl, toss the baby arugula with olive oil, lemon juice, salt, and pepper until well coated. Divide the dressed arugula among serving plates. Top with the cooked chicken meatballs.

5. Drizzle the whipped tahini over the meatballs and arugula. Garnish with additional grated Parmesan cheese or fresh herbs if desired.

Nutritional Information
Calories: 380 kcal
Carbohydrates: 12g
Protein: 25g
Fat: 27g
Saturated Fat: 5g
Cholesterol: 125mg
Sodium: 310mg
Fiber: 3g
Sugar: 1g

Shrimp with Green Beans

Prep Time: 15 minutes
Cook Time: 15 minutes
Servings: 4

Ingredients
- One pound of peeled and deveined large shrimp

- 1 pound fresh green beans, trimmed
- 2 tablespoons olive oil
- 3 cloves garlic, minced
- 1 teaspoon grated ginger
- 1 tablespoon low-sodium soy sauce
- 1 tablespoon oyster sauce (optional)
- 1/2 teaspoon sesame oil
- Salt and pepper to taste
- Red pepper flakes (optional for added heat)
- Sesame seeds for garnish (optional)

Procedure

1.   Rinse the shrimp under cold water and pat dry with paper towels. Sprinkle some salt and pepper on the shrimp for seasoning.

Trim the ends of the green beans and cut them into bite-sized pieces, if desired. Set aside.

2. A big skillet filled with one tablespoon of olive oil is heated to medium-high heat. When the green beans are brilliant green and just beginning to soften, add them to the skillet and simmer, turning periodically, for five to six minutes. After taking the green beans out of the skillet, set them aside.

3. Add the last tablespoon of olive oil to the same skillet. Once hot, add the minced garlic and grated ginger to the skillet. Sauté for 1-2 minutes, or until fragrant. Place the seasoned shrimp in a single layer within the skillet. Fry the shrimp for two to three minutes on each side, or until they are opaque and pink. Don't overcook the shrimp because that can make them tough

4. Return the cooked green beans to the skillet with the shrimp. Add the low-sodium soy sauce, oyster sauce (if using), sesame oil, and red pepper flakes (if desired). Stir well to coat the shrimp and green beans evenly with the sauce. Cook for a further one to two minutes, or until well heated.

5. Transfer the Shrimp with Green Beans to a serving platter or individual plates. Garnish with sesame seeds, if desired, for added flavor and texture. Serve hot as a main dish alongside cooked brown rice, quinoa, or cauliflower rice for a complete and balanced meal.

<u>**Notes**</u>

• Taste the shrimp and green beans before serving and adjust the seasoning if necessary. You can add more soy sauce for saltiness, a splash of lime juice for acidity, or a drizzle of honey or maple syrup for sweetness, depending on your taste preferences.

• Feel free to customize the recipe by using other vegetables in addition to or instead of green beans. Bell peppers, snap peas, broccoli, asparagus, or spinach would all work well in this dish. Keep in mind how long each veggie should cook for and make adjustments as necessary.

• If you prefer a lighter option, you can steam the green beans instead of sautéing them in olive oil. Simply place the trimmed green beans in a steamer basket over boiling water and steam for 3-4 minutes, or until tender-crisp.

• In addition to sesame seeds, you can garnish the dish with chopped fresh herbs such as cilantro, parsley, or green onions for added freshness and color. A sprinkle of toasted almonds or cashews would also add a nice crunch.

• It makes excellent leftovers and can be stored in an airtight container in the refrigerator for up to 2-3 days. To avoid drying out, reheat individual servings in the microwave or on the stovetop with a drop of water.

Nutritional Information
Calories: 210 kcal
Carbohydrates: 9g
Protein: 25g
Fat: 9g
Saturated Fat: 1.5g
Cholesterol: 190 mg
Sodium: 440mg
Fiber: 3g
Sugar: 3g

Cauliflower Tacos

Prep Time: 20 minutes

Ingredients
- Cut one medium head of cauliflower into florets.
- 2 tablespoons olive oil
- 1 teaspoon chili powder
- 1/2 teaspoon ground cumin
- 1/2 teaspoon smoked paprika
- 1/4 teaspoon garlic powder
- 1 ripe avocado
- 1/4 cup plain Greek yogurt (or dairy-free alternative)
- 2 tablespoons lime juice
- 1 clove garlic, minced
- Salt and pepper to taste
- Water

For Serving:
- 8 small corn or flour tortillas (use whole grain or low-carb tortillas for a healthier option)
- Shredded lettuce or cabbage
- Diced tomatoes
- Chopped fresh cilantro
- Lime wedges

Optional toppings: diced onions, sliced jalapeños, hot sauce

Procedure
1. Preheat your oven to 425°F (220°C). The baking sheet can be lightly oiled with olive oil or lined with parchment paper.

2. In a large mixing bowl, toss the cauliflower florets with olive oil, chili powder, ground cumin, smoked paprika, garlic powder, salt, and pepper until evenly coated.
- Arrange the seasoned cauliflower in a single layer on a parchment paper-lined baking sheet. Roast in the preheated oven for 20-25 minutes, or until the cauliflower is tender and golden brown, stirring halfway through cooking.

3. In a blender or food processor, combine the ripe avocado, Greek yogurt, lime juice, minced garlic, salt, and pepper. Blend until smooth and creamy. If the crema is too

thick, you can thin it out with a little water until you reach your desired consistency. Adjust the seasoning to taste.

4. While the cauliflower is roasting, warm the tortillas in a dry skillet or in the oven according to the package instructions. Keep the warm tortillas wrapped in a clean kitchen towel to prevent them from drying out.

5. To assemble the tacos, spoon some roasted cauliflower onto each warm tortilla. Top with shredded lettuce or cabbage, diced tomatoes, chopped fresh cilantro, and a drizzle of avocado crema.
    - Serve with lime wedges on the side for squeezing over the top. Add optional toppings such as diced onions, sliced jalapeños, or hot sauce for extra flavor and heat.

Notes
• Feel free to customize the seasoning for the roasted cauliflower to suit your taste preferences. You can add ingredients like onion powder, cayenne pepper, or chipotle powder for extra flavor and heat.

• You can also experiment with different cooking methods for the cauliflower. Instead of roasting, you can grill or sauté the cauliflower for a slightly different texture and flavor.

• Get creative with the toppings for the tacos. In addition to the suggested toppings, you can add sliced avocado, pickled red onions, black beans, corn kernels, or a drizzle of salsa verde or chipotle sauce.

• If you're following a gluten-free diet, make sure to use certified gluten-free tortillas. For a dairy-free option, you can use a dairy-free yogurt alternative or skip the avocado crema altogether and substitute with your favorite dairy-free sauce or dressing.

• You can prepare the roasted cauliflower and avocado crema ahead of time and store them in separate airtight containers in the refrigerator for up to 2-3 days. When ready to serve, simply reheat the cauliflower in the oven or microwave and assemble the tacos with the remaining ingredients.

• Serve with additional side dishes such as Mexican rice, refried beans, or a side salad for a complete and satisfying meal.

Nutritional Information
Calories: 280 kcal

Carbohydrates: 29g
Protein: 7g
Fat: 16g
Saturated Fat: 2.5g
Cholesterol: 0mg
Sodium: 320mg
Fiber: 7g
Sugar: 4g

Cream of Turkey & Wild Rice Soup

Prep Time: 15 minutes
Cook Time: 45 minutes
Servings: 6

Ingredients
- 1 tablespoon olive oil
- 1 onion, finely chopped
- 2 carrots, diced
- 2 celery stalks, diced
- 2 cloves garlic, minced
- 8 ounces cooked turkey breast, diced (skinless, boneless)
- 1/2 cup wild rice blend
- four cups of low-sodium turkey or chicken broth
- 1 teaspoon dried thyme
- 1/2 teaspoon dried sage
- Salt and pepper to taste
- cup unsweetened almond milk or low-fat milk
- 1/2 cup half-and-half or heavy cream (optional)
- 2 tablespoons cornstarch (optional, for thickening)
- Chopped fresh parsley for garnish

Procedure

1. In a big pot or Dutch oven, warm up the olive oil over medium heat. Add the chopped onion, diced carrots, and diced celery to the pot. Cook, stirring occasionally, for 5-6 minutes, or until the vegetables are softened and translucent.
- Cook the minced garlic in the pot for a further one to two minutes, or until it becomes aromatic.

2. Add the wild rice mixture and chopped turkey breast. To gently toast the rice, cook it for one to two minutes.
- Add the dried thyme, dry sage, low-sodium chicken or turkey broth, salt, and pepper. After bringing the mixture to a boil, turn down the heat. Cover and simmer for 30-35 minutes, or until the wild rice is tender and cooked through.

3. In a small bowl, whisk together the low-fat milk (or unsweetened almond milk) and cornstarch until smooth. Stir the mixture into the soup along with the half-and-half or heavy cream (if using). Cook for an additional 5-10 minutes, or until the soup has thickened slightly.

4. Taste the soup and adjust the seasoning with salt and pepper, if needed. If the soup is too thick, you can thin it out with additional broth or milk.
   - Ladle the Soup into bowls and garnish with chopped fresh parsley before serving.

<u>**Notes**</u>

• Feel free to customize the soup by adding additional vegetables such as diced potatoes, mushrooms, or spinach. You can also incorporate frozen peas or corn for added sweetness and texture.

• If you don't have cooked turkey breast on hand, you can use cooked chicken breast or turkey sausage instead. Simply dice the cooked meat or sausage and add it to the soup along with the other ingredients.

• If you don't have a wild rice blend, you can use regular wild rice or a combination of white and brown rice. Adjust the cooking time accordingly based on the type of rice used.

• For a creamier texture, you can blend a portion of the soup using an immersion blender or regular blender before adding the milk and cream. This will help thicken the soup and create a smoother consistency.

• In addition to chopped fresh parsley, you can garnish the soup with a dollop of Greek yogurt or sour cream, a sprinkle of grated Parmesan cheese, or a drizzle of extra virgin olive oil for added flavor and richness.

• You may prepare this soup in advance and keep it in the fridge for up to three or four days. Simply reheat individual portions in the microwave or on the stovetop with a splash of water or additional broth to thin out the soup if needed.

Nutritional Information
Calories: 220 kcal, Carbohydrates: 20g, Protein: 18g, Fat: 8g, Saturated Fat: 2g, Cholesterol: 40mg, Sodium: 400mg, Fiber: 2g, Sugar: 4g

Ginger-Tahini Oven-Baked Salmon & Vegetables

Prep Time: 15 minutes
Cook Time: 20 minutes
Servings: 4

Ingredients
- 1/4 cup tahini
- 2 tablespoons soy sauce (low-sodium)
- 1 tablespoon maple syrup or honey
- 1 tablespoon grated fresh ginger
- 2 cloves garlic, minced
- 1 tablespoon rice vinegar
- 1 tablespoon sesame oil
- 2 tablespoons water
- Salt and pepper to taste
- 6 ounce each of 4 salmon filets
- 4 cups mixed vegetables (such as broccoli florets, bell peppers, and carrots), chopped
- 2 tablespoons olive oil
- Sesame seeds and chopped green onions for garnish

Procedure

1. Preheat your oven to 400°F (200°C). Line a baking sheet with parchment paper or lightly grease it with olive oil.

2. In a small bowl, whisk together the tahini, soy sauce, maple syrup or honey, grated ginger, minced garlic, rice vinegar, sesame oil, water, salt, and pepper until smooth and well combined. Set aside.

3. Place the salmon filets in a shallow dish or resealable plastic bag. Pour half of the prepared ginger-tahini marinade over the salmon, reserving the remaining marinade for later use. Ensure that the salmon is evenly coated with the marinade. Cover and refrigerate for at least 15 minutes to allow the flavors to meld.

4. In a large mixing bowl, toss the chopped mixed vegetables with olive oil, salt, and pepper until well coated. Arrange the seasoned veggies on the baking sheet that has been preheated in a single layer.

5. Place the marinated salmon filets on the baking sheet alongside the seasoned vegetables. Bake in the preheated oven for 15-20 minutes, or until the salmon is cooked through and flakes easily with a fork, and the vegetables are tender and lightly browned around the edges.

6. Transfer the baked salmon filets and vegetables to serving plates. Drizzle the remaining ginger-tahini marinade over the salmon and vegetables.

7. Garnish with sesame seeds and chopped green onions for added flavor and presentation. Serve hot, alongside cooked quinoa, brown rice, or cauliflower rice for a complete and balanced meal.

Notes
• Feel free to customize the vegetables used in the recipe based on your preferences and what's available. You can use a variety of vegetables such as zucchini, cauliflower, Brussels sprouts, or green beans. Just make sure to adjust the cooking time accordingly for different vegetables.

• If you prefer, you can use other types of fish filets such as cod, halibut, or trout instead of salmon. Just remember to modify the cooking time for various vegetables accordingly

• For even more flavor, you can marinate the salmon filets for longer than 15 minutes. Marinating for up to 1 hour in the refrigerator will allow the flavors to penetrate the fish more deeply.

• In addition to sesame seeds and chopped green onions, you can garnish the dish with fresh herbs such as cilantro or parsley for added freshness and color. A squeeze of fresh lemon or lime juice over the finished dish can also brighten the flavors.

• This dish makes excellent leftovers and can be stored in an airtight container in the refrigerator for up to 2-3 days. Reheat individual portions in the microwave or in a skillet on the stovetop until warmed through.

• Serve with a side of steamed greens or a mixed green salad dressed with a simple vinaigrette for a complete and balanced meal.

Nutritional Information
Calories: 380 kcal, Carbohydrates: 14g, Protein: 30g, Fat: 24g, Saturated Fat: 4g, Cholesterol: 80mg, Sodium: 480mg, Fiber: 4g, Sugar: 6g

Pepper-Crusted Salmon with Garlic Chickpeas

Prep Time: 10 minutes
Cook Time: 20 minutes
Servings: 4

Ingredients
- 6 ounce each of 4 salmon filet
- 2 tablespoons olive oil
- 2 tablespoons coarsely ground black pepper
- 1 teaspoon smoked paprika
- 1 teaspoon garlic powder
- 1/2 teaspoon salt
- Two cans of (15 ounces each) chickpeas, rinsed and drained
- 2 tablespoons olive oil

- 4 cloves garlic, minced
- 1 teaspoon ground cumin
- 1 teaspoon ground coriander
- ¼ teaspoon of pepper
- Fresh lemon wedges for serving
- Chopped fresh parsley for garnish

Procedure

1. Preheat your oven to 400°F (200°C). Line a baking sheet with parchment paper or aluminum foil for easy cleanup.

2. Pat the salmon filets dry with paper towels and place them on the prepared baking sheet. Drizzle the salmon filets with olive oil and use your hands to rub the oil evenly over the surface of each filet. In a small bowl, combine the coarsely ground black pepper, smoked paprika, garlic powder, and salt. Sprinkle the pepper mixture evenly over the salmon filets, pressing gently to adhere.

3. Place the seasoned salmon filets in the preheated oven and roast for 12-15 minutes, or until the salmon is cooked through and flakes easily with a fork. The thickness of the filets will determine how long they take to cook. If using skin-on salmon, the skin should be crisp and golden brown.

4. While the salmon is roasting, heat olive oil in a large skillet over medium heat. Add the minced garlic to the skillet and sauté for 1-2 minutes, or until fragrant. Add the drained and rinsed chickpeas to the skillet, along with ground cumin, ground coriander, salt, and pepper. Cook, stirring occasionally, for 5-7 minutes, or until the chickpeas are heated through and slightly crispy on the outside.

5. Divide the roasted salmon filets and garlic chickpeas among serving plates.
   - Garnish with chopped fresh parsley and serve with fresh lemon wedges on the side for squeezing over the salmon.
   - Enjoy a delicious and nutritious meal!

<u>Notes</u>

• Consider serving the salmon and chickpeas with a side of roasted or steamed vegetables, such as broccoli, asparagus, or green beans, to add more fiber, vitamins, and minerals to the meal.

• Instead of serving the salmon filets whole, you can flake the cooked salmon and toss it with the garlic chickpeas to create a flavorful and protein-packed salad. Serve the salad over a bed of mixed greens for a light and refreshing meal.

• Adjust the amount of black pepper and spices used in the pepper crust according to your taste preferences. If you prefer a milder flavor, you can reduce the amount of black pepper or omit it altogether.

• Store any leftover salmon and garlic chickpeas in separate airtight containers in the refrigerator for up to 2-3 days. Reheat individual portions in the microwave or in a skillet on the stovetop until warmed through.

• Feel free to use other types of salmon filets such as sockeye, coho, or king salmon based on availability and personal preference. Opt for wild-caught salmon whenever possible for its superior flavor and nutritional profile.

• In addition to chopped parsley, you can garnish the dish with a sprinkle of lemon zest, chopped fresh dill, or thinly sliced green onions for added freshness and visual appeal.

Nutritional Information
Calories: 450 kcal, Carbohydrates: 28g, Protein: 30g, Fat: 24g, Saturated Fat: 3.5g, Cholesterol: 75mg, Sodium: 570mg, Fiber: 8g, Sugar: 1g.

APPETIZER AND SNACK RECIPES

Cheesy Kale Chips

Prep Time: 10 minutes
Cook Time: 20-25 minutes
Servings: 4

Ingredients
- 1 large bunch of kale (about 10-12 cups), washed and dried
- 2 tablespoons olive oil
- 1/4 cup nutritional yeast
- 1 teaspoon garlic powder
- 1/2 teaspoon onion powder
- 1/2 teaspoon paprika
- 1/4 teaspoon salt, or to taste
- Cooking spray or additional olive oil (for greasing)

Procedure
1. Preheat the oven to 300°F (150°C).
 - Use silicone baking mats or parchment paper to line two large baking sheets. After giving the kale leaves a good wash in cold water, pat them dry with paper towels or a fresh kitchen towel. Tear the kale leaves into bite-sized pieces after removing the stiff stems.

2.   In a small bowl, combine the olive oil, nutritional yeast, garlic powder, onion powder, paprika, and salt. Stir well to create a cheesy seasoning mixture.
   - In a large mixing bowl, Place the kale pieces. Drizzle the seasoned olive oil mixture over the kale leaves.

3. Using your hands, gently massage the seasoned olive oil mixture into the kale leaves, ensuring that each leaf is evenly coated with the seasoning.

4. Make sure the kale leaves do not overlap when you arrange them in a single layer on the baking sheets.

5. Place the baking sheets in the preheated oven and bake the kale chips for 20-25 minutes, or until the edges are crisp and the kale leaves are lightly golden brown. As the baking time comes to a finish, keep a watch on them to avoid burning.

6. Remove from the oven and let them cool on the baking sheets for a few minutes.
   - Once cooled, transfer the kale chips to a serving bowl or plate.

Nutritional Information
- Per serving (1/4 of the recipe): Calories: 120 kcal, Carbohydrates: 8g, Protein: 5g, Fat: 8g, Saturated Fat: 1g, Cholesterol: 0mg, Sodium: 160mg, Fiber: 3g, Sugar: 1g

Tuna Cucumber Bites

Prep Time: 15 minutes
Servings: 12 bites

Ingredients
- 1 can (5 ounces) tuna in water, drained
- 1/4 cup Greek yogurt
- 1 tablespoon lemon juice
- 2 tablespoons finely chopped red onion
- 2 tablespoons finely chopped celery
- 1 tablespoon chopped fresh parsley
- Salt and pepper to taste
- 1 large cucumber, washed and cut into thick slices
Optional toppings: cherry tomatoes, sliced olives, chopped bell peppers, etc.

Procedure
1. Start by draining the water or oil from the canned tuna. You can use a fork to press out any excess liquid.

- In a mixing bowl, combine the drained tuna with Greek yogurt, lemon juice, finely chopped red onion, celery, and fresh parsley. These ingredients add flavor and texture to the tuna mixture.

   - Add Salt and Pepper to the mixture with salt and pepper to taste. Be mindful of the salt content, especially if you're using canned tuna, which may already be salty.

2. Depending on your preference, you can adjust the consistency of the tuna mixture. If you prefer a creamier texture, you can add more Greek yogurt. If you prefer a tangier flavor, you can add more lemon juice.

3. Wash the cucumber thoroughly under cold water to remove any dirt or debris. You can peel the cucumber if desired, or leave the skin on for added fiber and texture.

   - Use a sharp knife to slice the cucumber into thick rounds, about 1/2 inch thick. These will serve as the base for the tuna mixture.

4. Once the tuna mixture is ready, place a spoonful of the mixture on top of each cucumber slice. Use the back of the spoon to spread the mixture evenly over the surface of the cucumber.

5. To enhance the flavor and presentation of the tuna cucumber bites, you can add optional toppings such as halved cherry tomatoes, sliced olives, chopped bell peppers, or fresh herbs like dill or chives.

   - These toppings not only add color and texture but also provide additional nutrients and flavor to the dish.

6. Arrange the prepared tuna cucumber bites on a serving platter or plate.

   - These bites are best enjoyed fresh but can be stored in the refrigerator for a few hours before serving.

Nutritional Information
- Per serving (1 cucumber bite, without optional toppings): Calories: 25 kcal, Carbohydrates: 1g, Protein: 4g, Fat: 1g, Saturated Fat: 0g, Cholesterol: 5mg, Sodium: 70mg, Fiber: 0g, Sugar: 0g

Pumpkin Goat Cheese Puff Pastry Rolls

Prep Time: 20 minutes

Cook Time: 20 minutes

Servings: 12 rolls

Ingredients
- 1 sheet of puff pastry, thawed according to package instructions
- 1/2 cup pumpkin puree (unsweetened)
- 4 ounces goat cheese, softened
- 1 tablespoon honey (optional)
- 1/4 teaspoon ground cinnamon
- 1/4 teaspoon ground nutmeg
- Salt and pepper to taste
- 1 egg, beaten (for egg wash)
- Poppy or sesame seeds (optional, for garnishing)

Procedure
1. Preheat your oven to 400°F (200°C). Use silicone baking mats or parchment paper to line two large baking sheets

2. In a mixing bowl, combine the pumpkin puree, softened goat cheese, honey (if using), ground cinnamon, ground nutmeg, salt, and pepper. Taste and adjust the seasoning to your desired level. The honey adds a touch of sweetness, but you can omit it if you prefer a less sweet filling.

3. On a lightly floured surface, unfold the thawed puff pastry sheet. Use a rolling pin to gently roll out the pastry sheet to even out any creases and slightly increase its size.

4. Spread the pumpkin-goat cheese mixture evenly over the surface of the puff pastry sheet, leaving a small border along one of the longer edges. This border will help seal the rolls later.

5. Starting from the long edge opposite the border, carefully roll up the puff pastry sheet into a tight log. Use your fingers to gently press the border onto the roll to seal it.

6. Using a sharp knife, slice the rolled-up pastry into approximately 12 equal-sized pieces. Aim for around one inch thick pieces. You can lightly mark the pastry with a knife before cutting to ensure even slices.

7. Place the sliced rolls on the prepared baking sheet, spacing them evenly apart. Leave some room between the rolls as they will expand slightly during baking.

8. In a small bowl, beat the egg until well combined. Use a pastry brush to lightly brush the tops of the pastry rolls with the beaten egg. This will give them a shiny and golden finish as they bake.

9. If desired, sprinkle sesame seeds, poppy seeds, or finely chopped herbs over the tops of the rolls for added flavor and visual appeal. Press them gently into the pastry to ensure they adhere.

10. Transfer the baking sheet to the preheated oven and bake the pumpkin goat cheese puff pastry rolls for about 20 minutes, or until they are puffed up and golden brown. Keep an eye on them towards the end of the baking time to prevent over-browning.

11. Once baked, remove the rolls from the oven and allow them to cool slightly on the baking sheet for a few minutes before transferring them to a wire rack to cool completely.

Nutritional Information
- Per serving (1 roll): Calories: 160 kcal, Carbohydrates: 11g, Protein: 4g, Fat: 11g, Saturated Fat: 5g, Cholesterol: 30mg, Sodium: 140mg, Fiber: 1g, Sugar: 2g

Edamame

Prep Time: 5 minutes
Cook Time: 5-7 minutes
Servings: 4

Ingredients
- 2 cups frozen edamame in pods
- Water
- Salt (optional, for seasoning)

Procedure

1. If using frozen edamame, remove the desired amount from the package and place it in a colander. Rinse the edamame under cold water to thaw it slightly. Alternatively, you can let it sit at room temperature for a few minutes until it softens slightly.

2. Fill a medium-sized pot with water and bring it to a rolling boil over high heat. Adding salt to the water is optional but can enhance the flavor of the edamame.

3. While waiting for the water to boil, inspect the edamame pods for any debris or damaged pods. Remove any stems or stray pieces.

4. Once the water is boiling, carefully add the edamame pods to the pot. Make sure the pods are submerged in the water.
    - Allow the edamame to cook for 5-7 minutes, or until they are tender. The pods will turn a brighter green color when they are cooked.

5. To check if the edamame is cooked to your liking, carefully remove one pod from the boiling water using tongs or a slotted spoon. Allow it to cool slightly, then peel open the pod and taste one of the beans. The beans should be tender but still have a slight bite to them.

6. Once the edamame is cooked to perfection, carefully drain them in a colander and shake off any excess water. You can also rinse them briefly under cold water to stop the cooking process and cool them down.
    - Placed the cooked edamame in a bowl for serving
If desired, sprinkle them with a pinch of salt while they are still warm. You can also experiment with other seasonings such as garlic powder, chili flakes, or sesame seeds for added flavor.

7. Serve immediately as a nutritious snack or side dish. You can eat them warm, hot, or at room temperature.
    - To eat, simply squeeze the pod gently between your teeth to release the beans. Discard the empty pod and enjoy the delicious, tender beans inside.

Baked Sweet Potato Coins

Prep Time: 10 minutes
Cook Time: 25-30 minutes
Servings: 4

Ingredients
- 2 medium sweet potatoes, scrubbed clean
- 2 tablespoons olive oil
- 1 teaspoon smoked paprika
- 1/2 teaspoon garlic powder
- 1/2 teaspoon onion powder
- 1/4 teaspoon salt, or to taste
- 1/4 teaspoon black pepper, or to taste

Procedure
1. Preheat your oven to 400°F (200°C). This ensures that the oven is fully heated and ready for baking when you're done preparing the sweet potato coins.

2. Under running water, give the sweet potatoes a good wash to get rid of any dirt or debris. If required, use a vegetable scrubber. Using a fresh kitchen towel, pat them dry. Using a sharp knife, carefully cut the sweet potatoes into rounds that are uniformly 1/4 inch thick. To achieve even cooking, try to make the slices as uniform as you can.

3. In a large mixing bowl, combine the sweet potato slices with olive oil, smoked paprika, garlic powder, onion powder, salt, and black pepper. The olive oil helps the seasoning adhere to the sweet potatoes and promotes crispiness during baking.
   - Use clean hands or a spoon to toss the sweet potato slices until they are evenly coated with the seasoning mixture. Ensure that each slice is well coated for maximum flavor.

4. Line a baking sheet with parchment paper or aluminum foil for easy cleanup. Arrange the seasoned sweet potato coins in a single layer on the prepared baking sheet, making sure they are evenly spaced and not overlapping. This facilitates even cooking and appropriate air movement.

- If you have a large batch of sweet potatoes, you may need to use multiple baking sheets or bake them in batches to avoid overcrowding.

5. Place the baking sheet in the preheated oven and bake the sweet potato coins for 25-30 minutes, flipping them halfway through the cooking time. Flipping them ensures that both sides cook evenly and develop a crispy exterior.
   - Keep an eye on the sweet potato coins towards the end of the baking time to prevent burning. They should be golden brown and crispy on the outside, and tender on the inside when done.

6. Once the sweet potato coins are baked to perfection, remove them from the oven and transfer them to a serving platter or plate.
   - If desired, garnish the sweet potato coins with chopped fresh herbs such as parsley or thyme for a burst of freshness and flavor.
   - Serve hot as a delicious side dish or snack option alongside your favorite dipping sauce or condiment.

Nutritional Information
- Per serving (about 1/2 cup): Calories: 120 kcal, Carbohydrates: 18g, Protein: 2g, Fat: 5g, Saturated Fat: 1g, Cholesterol: 0mg, Sodium: 160mg, Fiber: 3g, Sugar: 4g

Apple-Raspberry Granola Skillet

Prep Time: 10 minutes
Cook Time: 20 minutes
Servings: 4

Ingredients
- Two medium apples, peeled and sliced thinly
- 1 cup fresh raspberries
- Two tablespoons of coconut oil or unsalted butter
- 2 tablespoons honey or maple syrup
- 1 teaspoon ground cinnamon
- 1/4 teaspoon ground nutmeg
- 1/4 teaspoon vanilla extract

- 1 cup granola (choose a low-sugar or sugar-free option for a diabetic-friendly version)
Optional toppings: Greek yogurt, chopped nuts, additional berries

Procedure

1. Preheat your oven to 375°F (190°C). This ensures that the oven is fully heated and ready for baking when you're done preparing the skillet.

2. Core the apples and thinly slice them. You can leave the skin on for added fiber and texture, or peel them if preferred. Rinse the raspberries under cold water and pat them dry with a paper towel to remove any excess moisture.
   - In a large mixing bowl, combine the thinly sliced apples and fresh raspberries. Gently toss to mix and evenly distribute the fruits.

3. In a large ovenproof skillet or frying pan, melt the unsalted butter or coconut oil over medium heat. Swirl the pan to coat the bottom evenly with the melted fat.

4. Once the butter is melted and the skillet is hot, add the mixed apples and raspberries to the skillet. To make sure they cook through, spread them out into an even layer.
   - Cook the fruit for about 5-7 minutes, stirring occasionally with a spatula or wooden spoon. The fruit should start to soften and release their juices, creating a deliciously fragrant mixture.

5. Drizzle the honey or maple syrup over the cooked fruit in the skillet. Sprinkle ground cinnamon, ground nutmeg, and vanilla extract over the mixture. Stir well to coat the fruit evenly with the sweeteners and spices.
   - Adjust the amount of sweeteners and spices according to your taste preferences. You can also omit the sweeteners entirely if the fruit is naturally sweet enough for your liking.

6. Sprinkle the granola evenly over the top of the fruit mixture in the skillet. Use a spatula or spoon to gently press the granola into the fruit, ensuring that it adheres and forms a crunchy topping.

7. Carefully transfer the skillet to the preheated oven and bake for 10-12 minutes, or until the granola is golden brown and crisp. Keep an eye on the skillet towards the end of the baking time to prevent burning.

8.   Once it is baked to perfection, remove it from the oven and let it cool slightly before serving.

   - Serve the skillet hot, either on its own or topped with Greek yogurt, chopped nuts, or additional berries for added flavor and texture.

Nutritional Information

- Per serving (1/4 of the recipe): Calories: 220 kcal, Carbohydrates: 34g, Protein: 3g, Fat: 9g, Saturated Fat: 4g, Cholesterol: 15mg, Sodium: 40mg, Fiber: 6g, Sugar: 20g

BEAN AND PASTA RECIPES

Mango & Kale Wheat Berry Salad

Prep Time: 15 minutes
Cook Time: 45 minutes (for wheat berries)
Servings: 4

Ingredients
- 1 cup wheat berries
- 2 cups water or low-sodium vegetable broth
- One can (15 ounces) of black beans rinsed and drained
- 1 ripe mango, diced
- 2 cups kale, chopped
- 1/4 cup red onion, finely chopped
- 1/4 cup fresh cilantro, chopped
- 2 tablespoons lime juice
- 2 tablespoons olive oil
- One teaspoon honey or maple syrup optional
- Salt and pepper to taste

Optional garnishes include feta cheese crumbles, pumpkin seeds, and avocado slices.

Procedure

1. Rinse the wheat berries under cold water until the water runs clear. In a medium saucepan, combine the rinsed wheat berries with water or vegetable broth. Bring to a boil over high heat.

   - Once boiling, reduce the heat to low, cover, and simmer for about 45-50 minutes, or until the wheat berries are tender but still chewy. Drain any excess liquid and let the wheat berries cool slightly.

2. In a large mixing bowl, combine the cooked wheat berries, black beans, diced mango, chopped kale, finely chopped red onion, and chopped cilantro. Toss gently to mix.

3. In a small bowl, whisk together the lime juice, olive oil, honey or maple syrup (if using), salt, and pepper until well combined. Adjust the seasoning to taste.

4. Pour the dressing over the salad mixture in the large bowl. Gently toss to ensure that the dressing coats every ingredient equally. Make sure the salad is well combined and coated with the dressing.

5. Transfer to a serving dish or individual bowls. If desired, top with avocado slices, pumpkin seeds, or crumbled feta cheese for added flavor and texture.
   - Serve the salad immediately as a nutritious and satisfying meal, or refrigerate it for 1-2 hours to allow the flavors to meld before serving.

Nutritional Information
- Per serving (about 1 1/2 cups): Calories: 320 kcal, Carbohydrates: 53g, Protein: 10g, Fat: 9g, Saturated Fat: 1g, Cholesterol: 0mg, Sodium: 200mg, Fiber: 10g, Sugar: 9g

Zucchini Pasta with Lemon and Asparagus

Prep Time: 15 minutes
Cook Time: 10 minutes
Servings: 4

Ingredients
- 4 medium zucchini
- 1 bunch asparagus, tough ends trimmed and cut into bite-sized pieces
- 2 cloves garlic, minced
- Zest and juice of 1 lemon
- 2 tablespoons olive oil
- Salt and pepper to taste
Optional garnishes grated Parmesan cheese, chopped fresh herbs (such as parsley or basil), red pepper flakes

Procedure

1. Wash the zucchini thoroughly under running water to remove any dirt or debris. Cut off the zucchini's ends.

   - Using a spiralizer, spiralize the zucchini into long, thin strands resembling pasta noodles. Alternatively, if you don't have a spiralizer, you can use a vegetable peeler to create long, thin strips of zucchini. Set the zucchini noodles aside.

2. Wash the asparagus spears under cold water and pat them dry with a paper towel. Trim off the tough ends of the asparagus and discard them.
   - Cut the asparagus spears into bite-sized pieces, about 1-inch in length.
   - One tablespoon of olive oil should be heated over medium heat in a big skillet. Once the garlic is fragrant, add it to the skillet and mince it. Cook for one minute.

3. Add the asparagus pieces to the skillet and sauté for 3-4 minutes, stirring occasionally, until they are tender-crisp. Add salt and pepper.
- Once the asparagus is cooked, transfer it to a plate and set it aside.

4. In the same skillet, add the remaining tablespoon of olive oil. Add the zucchini noodles to the skillet and sauté them for 2-3 minutes, stirring occasionally, until they are just tender. Be careful not to overcook the zucchini, as it can become mushy.
   - Return the cooked asparagus to the skillet with the zucchini noodles. Add the lemon zest and lemon juice to the skillet, tossing everything together gently to combine.
   - Taste the zucchini pasta and adjust the seasoning with salt and pepper as needed.

5. Transfer to serving plates or bowls.
   - If desired, garnish each serving with grated Parmesan cheese, chopped fresh herbs such as parsley or basil, and a sprinkle of red pepper flakes for added flavor and texture.

Nutritional Information
- Per serving (about 1 1/2 cups Calories: 110 kcal, Carbohydrates: 10g, Protein: 4g, Fat: 7g, Saturated Fat: 1g, Cholesterol: 0mg, Sodium: 10mg, Fiber: 4g, Sugar: 5g

Sesame-Garlic Beef & Broccoli with Whole-Wheat Noodles

Prep Time: 15 minutes
Cook Time: 15 minutes
Servings:4

Ingredients
- 8 ounces whole-wheat spaghetti or noodles
- 1 pound flank steak, thinly sliced against the grain
- 2 cups broccoli florets
- 3 cloves garlic, minced
- 2 tablespoons low-sodium soy sauce
- 1 tablespoon sesame oil
- 1 tablespoon honey or maple syrup
- 1 tablespoon rice vinegar
- 1 teaspoon cornstarch (optional, for thickening)
- 2 tablespoons sesame seeds
- Two thinly sliced onion for garnish
- Salt and pepper to taste
- Optional garnish: red pepper flakes

Procedure
1.   Heat a big saucepan of salted water till it boils. After adding the whole-wheat spaghetti or noodles, cook them as directed on the package until they are al dente. After draining, place the noodles aside.

2. In a small bowl, whisk together the minced garlic, low-sodium soy sauce, sesame oil, honey or maple syrup, and rice vinegar to make the sauce. Set aside. In a large saucepan, warm up olive oil in high-medium heat. Add the thinly sliced flank steak to the skillet and season with salt and pepper to taste.

- Cook the beef for 2-3 minutes, stirring occasionally, until it is browned and cooked through. Set the beef aside after you have removed it from the skillet.

- In the same skillet, add the broccoli florets and cook for 3-4 minutes, or until they are bright green and slightly tender. If needed, you can add a splash of water to the skillet to help steam the broccoli.

3. Return the cooked beef to the skillet with the broccoli. Pour the prepared sauce over the beef and broccoli mixture in the skillet. Toss everything together gently to coat the beef and broccoli evenly with the sauce.
   - If desired, you can thicken the sauce by mixing 1 teaspoon of cornstarch with 1 tablespoon of water in a small bowl. Stir thoroughly after adding the cornstarch mixture to the skillet. Cook for an additional minute, or until the sauce has thickened slightly.

4. Divide among serving plates or bowls. Top the noodles with the Sesame-Garlic Beef & Broccoli mixture from the skillet.
   - Garnish each serving with sesame seeds and thinly sliced green onions. If desired, sprinkle with red pepper flakes for added heat.
   - Serve the dish immediately as a delicious and satisfying meal.

Notes
• Feel free to adjust the sauce to suit your taste preferences. You can add more or less honey or soy sauce depending on your preference for sweetness or saltiness.

• While broccoli is traditional in this dish, you can also add other vegetables such as bell peppers, snap peas, or carrots for extra color and nutrients.

• Garnish the dish with additional toppings such as crushed peanuts, chopped cilantro, or a squeeze of lime juice for added flavor and freshness.

• You can prepare the sauce and slice the beef and vegetables ahead of time to save time on busy weeknights. Store them separately in the refrigerator and cook everything together when ready to serve.

• For a complete meal, consider serving this dish with a side of steamed edamame, a fresh green salad, or a side of kimchi for added flavor and variety.

Nutritional Information
- Per serving (1/4 of the recipe): Calories: 420 kcal, Carbohydrates: 45g, Protein: 32g, Fat: 14g, Saturated Fat: 4g, Cholesterol: 60mg, Sodium: 550mg, Fiber: 8g, Sugar: 5g

Zesty Shrimp & Black Bean Salad

Prep Time: 15 minutes
Cook Time: 10 minutes
Servings: 4

Ingredients
- 1 pound shrimp, peeled and deveined
- One can of (15 ounces) black beans rinsed and drained
- 1 cup cherry tomatoes, halved
- 1/2 red onion, finely chopped
- 1/4 cup fresh cilantro, chopped
- 1 avocado, diced
- 2 tablespoons lime juice
- 2 tablespoons olive oil
- 1 teaspoon ground cumin
- 1/2 teaspoon chili powder
- Salt and pepper to taste
- **Optional garnishes**: sliced jalapeños, diced bell peppers, crumbled feta cheese

Procedure

1. Start by peeling and deveining a shrimp, if they haven't been done already. After giving them a quick rinse in cold water, blot dry with paper towels. Season the shrimp with salt, pepper, ground cumin, and chili powder. Toss them gently to ensure even seasoning.

2. Heat a large skillet over medium-high heat. Drizzle the skillet with olive oil.
   - Once the skillet is hot, add the seasoned shrimp in a single layer, making sure not to overcrowd the pan.
Shrimp should be cooked for two to three minutes on each side, or until they are opaque and pink. They might turn tough if they are overcooked.
   - Once cooked, remove the shrimp from the skillet and transfer them to a plate lined with paper towels to drain any excess oil. Set them aside.

3. While the shrimp are cooking, prepare the other salad ingredients. Drain and rinse the black beans under cold water to remove any excess sodium. Put them in a large mixing bowl. Wash and halve the cherry tomatoes, finely chop the red onion, and chop the fresh cilantro. Combine them with the black beans in the mixing basin.
   - Dice the avocado and add it to the mixing bowl as well. Toss the ingredients gently to combine.

4. In a small bowl, whisk together the lime juice, olive oil, and a pinch of salt and pepper until well combined. Adjust the seasoning to taste.

5. Pour the dressing over the salad ingredients in the mixing bowl. Use salad tongs or a large spoon to toss everything together gently, ensuring that all the ingredients are evenly coated with the dressing.
   - Add the cooked shrimp to the salad mixture in the bowl. Gently toss to combine, being careful not to break apart the shrimp.

6. Transfer to a serving dish or individual plates.
   - Garnish the salad with sliced jalapeños, diced bell peppers, or crumbled feta cheese, if desired.
   - Serve the salad immediately as a light and refreshing meal.

Nutritional Information
- Per serving (about 1 1/2 cups): Calories: 320 kcal, Carbohydrates: 22g, Protein: 25g, Fat: 16g, Saturated Fat: 2g, Cholesterol: 180mg, Sodium: 300mg, Fiber: 8g, Sugar: 2g

Spaghetti Squash Bolognese

Prep Time: 15 minutes
Cook Time: 1 hour
Servings: 4

Ingredients
- 1 medium spaghetti squash

- 1 tablespoon olive oil
- 1 small onion, finely chopped
- 2 cloves garlic, minced
- 1 pound lean ground beef (or ground turkey)
- 1 can (14.5 ounces) diced tomatoes
- 1 can (6 ounces) tomato paste
- 1 teaspoon dried oregano
- 1 teaspoon dried basil
- Salt and pepper to taste
- Grated Parmesan cheese for garnish
- Fresh basil leaves for garnish

Procedure

1. Preheat your oven to 400°F (200°C). Using a sharp knife, carefully cut the spaghetti squash in half lengthwise. Scoop out the stringy pulp and seeds from the center of each half using a spoon.

- Drizzle the cut sides of the squash halves with olive oil and season with salt and pepper. Rub the oil and seasonings evenly over the surface of the squash.

- Squash halves should be placed, cut side down, on a baking sheet covered with aluminum foil or parchment paper.

- Roast the squash in the preheated oven for 40-45 minutes, or until the flesh is tender and easily pierced with a fork.

- Once cooked, remove the squash from the oven and let it cool slightly before handling.

2. While the squash is roasting, prepare the bolognese sauce.

- In a large saucepan, warm up olive oil over medium heat. Add the chopped onion and minced garlic, and sauté until softened and translucent, about 5 minutes.

- Add the ground beef to the skillet and cook, breaking it apart with a spoon, until browned and cooked through.

- Stir in the diced tomatoes, tomato paste, dried oregano, dried basil, and a pinch of salt and pepper. Incorporate all the ingredients well

- After bringing the sauce to a simmer, turn down the heat. Let the sauce simmer gently for 15-20 minutes, stirring occasionally, to allow the flavors to meld and the sauce to thicken. If the sauce becomes too thick, you can add a splash of water or beef broth to loosen it up.

3. Once the spaghetti squash is cooked and slightly cooled, use a fork to scrape the flesh into spaghetti-like strands.

- Divide the spaghetti squash strands among serving plates or bowls.

  - Spoon the bolognese sauce over the spaghetti squash, dividing it evenly among the servings.

  - Garnish each serving with grated Parmesan cheese and fresh basil leaves, if desired.

  - Serve immediately, and enjoy

Nutritional Information

- Per serving (1/4 of the recipe): Calories: 350 kcal, Carbohydrates: 24g, Protein: 25g, Fat: 18g, Saturated Fat: 6g, Cholesterol: 70mg, Sodium: 600mg, Fiber: 6g, Sugar: 10g

Caribbean Tofu with Black Beans and Rice

Prep Time: 15 minutes
Cook Time: 30 minutes
Servings: 4

For the Caribbean Tofu:

- One block (fourteen ounces) of extra-firm, pressed, and cubed tofu

- 2 tablespoons olive oil

- 2 cloves garlic, minced

- 1 teaspoon ground cumin

- 1 teaspoon ground coriander

- 1 teaspoon smoked paprika

- 1/2 teaspoon ground turmeric

- 1/2 teaspoon chili powder

- 1/4 teaspoon cayenne (optional; add more heat if desired)

- Salt and pepper to taste

- Juice of 1 lime

- Two teaspoons of freshly chopped cilantro (for garnish)

Black beans

- One can of (15 ounces) black beans rinsed and drained

- 1/2 onion, finely chopped

- 1 bell pepper, diced

- 2 cloves garlic, minced
- 1 teaspoon ground cumin
- 1 teaspoon ground coriander
- 1 tablespoon olive oil
- 1/4 cup vegetable broth or water

For the Rice:
- 1 cup long-grain white rice
- 2 cups water
- 1 tablespoon olive oil
- Salt to taste

Procedure

1. To begin, press the tofu to squeeze off extra liquid. Sandwich the tofu between two clean kitchen towels or paper towels, then set something heavy (such a plate or skillet filled with weights) on top. Give the tofu a minimum of fifteen minutes to press.

   - Once pressed, cut the tofu into cubes and set aside.

   - In a large bowl, combine the cubed tofu with minced garlic, ground cumin, ground coriander, smoked paprika, ground turmeric, chili powder, cayenne pepper (if using), salt, pepper, and the juice of one lime. Toss until the tofu is evenly coated with the spices and lime juice.

2. In a big skillet set over medium-high heat, warm up the olive oil. Don't overcrowd the skillet by adding the seasoned tofu cubes in a single layer. Tofu should be cooked for 3–4 minutes on each side, or until crispy and golden brown. After taking the tofu out of the skillet, set it aside.

3. In the same skillet, heat another tablespoon of olive oil over medium heat. Add the finely chopped onion and diced bell pepper to the skillet, and sauté until softened, about 5 minutes.

   - When aromatic, add the minced garlic to the skillet and cook for an additional minute.

   - Stir in the drained and rinsed black beans, ground cumin, ground coriander, salt, and pepper. Cook for 2-3 minutes, stirring occasionally.

   - Add vegetable broth or water to the skillet, and let the beans simmer for another 5-7 minutes, or until heated through and the flavors are well combined.

4. In a medium saucepan, combine the long-grain white rice, water, olive oil, and salt. Bring to a boil over high heat.

- Once boiling, reduce the heat to low, cover, and simmer for 18-20 minutes, or until the rice is tender and all the water is absorbed. Before serving, use a fork to fluff the rice

5. To serve, divide the cooked rice among serving plates or bowls. Top each serving with a portion of the Caribbean tofu and black beans.
    - Garnish with chopped fresh cilantro.
    - Serve hot and enjoy!

Nutritional Information
- *Per serving (1/4 of the recipe):* Calories: 420 kcal, Carbohydrates: 57g, Protein: 18g, Fat: 15g, Saturated Fat: 2g, Cholesterol: 0mg, Sodium: 480mg, Fiber: 9g, Sugar: 2g

Chicken, Pasta, and Spinach Soup

Prep Time: 15 minutes
Cook Time: 25 minutes
Servings: 6

Ingredients
- 1 tablespoon olive oil
- 1 onion, diced
- 2 cloves garlic, minced
- 2 carrots, peeled and sliced
- 2 celery stalks, sliced
- 6 cups low-sodium chicken broth
- 2 cups cooked shredded chicken breast
- 1 cup uncooked whole grain pasta (such as penne or fusilli)
- 2 cups fresh baby spinach leaves
- 1 teaspoon dried thyme
- Salt and pepper to taste
- Grated Parmesan cheese for serving (optional)

Procedure

1. In a big pot, warm up the olive oil over medium heat. Add diced onion and minced garlic, and sauté until softened and fragrant, about 2-3 minutes.
   - Add sliced carrots and celery to the pot, and continue to sauté for another 3-4 minutes, until the vegetables begin to soften.

2. Pour in the low-sodium chicken broth, and bring the mixture to a boil.
   - Once boiling, reduce the heat to low and add the cooked shredded chicken breast to the pot. To let the flavors combine, boil the soup for ten minutes.

3. While the soup is simmering, cook the uncooked whole grain pasta separately according to the package instructions until al dente. Drain and set aside.

4. Add the cooked pasta to the soup pot, stirring gently to combine. Let the soup simmer for an additional 5 minutes to allow the pasta to absorb some of the broth and flavors.
   - Stir in dried thyme, and season with salt and pepper to taste.

5. Just before serving, add fresh baby spinach leaves to the soup pot. Stir until the spinach wilts and becomes tender, about 1-2 minutes.

6.   If desired, garnish each serving with a sprinkle of grated Parmesan cheese for added flavor.
   - Serve hot and enjoy!

<u>**Notes**</u>
• You can save time by using pre-cooked shredded chicken, such as rotisserie chicken, or leftover cooked chicken from a previous meal.

• To make the soup even heartier, consider adding additional vegetables such as diced bell peppers, diced zucchini, or chopped kale.

• If you prefer a thicker soup, you can add a tablespoon of cornstarch mixed with water to the soup during the last few minutes of cooking, stirring until thickened.

• You can add herbs like rosemary or parsley for additional flavor.

• For up to three to four days, leftovers can be kept in the refrigerator in an airtight container. Before serving, reheat the soup slowly over the stove or in the microwave.

Nutritional Information

-Per serving (1/6 of the recipe): Calories: 240 kcal, Carbohydrates: 20g, Protein: 20g, Fat: 8g, Saturated Fat: 1.5g, Cholesterol: 40mg, Sodium: 350mg, Fiber: 3g, Sugar: 3g

Spinach & Black Bean Burritos

Prep Time: 15 minutes
Cook Time: 15 minutes
Servings: 4

For the Filling:
- 1 tablespoon olive oil
- 1 small onion, diced
- 2 cloves garlic, minced
- 1 teaspoon ground cumin
- 1 teaspoon chili powder
- 1/2 teaspoon smoked paprika
- One can of (15 ounces) black beans rinsed and drained
- 2 cups fresh spinach leaves, chopped
- Salt and pepper to taste

For Assembling:
- 4 whole wheat tortillas
- 1 cup shredded reduced-fat cheese (such as cheddar or Monterey Jack)
- Salsa, avocado, Greek yogurt, or other desired toppings

Procedure

1.   In a big pot, warm up the olive oil over medium heat. Add diced onion and minced garlic, and sauté until softened and fragrant, about 2-3 minutes.

   - Add ground cumin, chili powder, and smoked paprika to the skillet, and stir to coat the onions and garlic with the spices.

- Add drained and rinsed black beans to the skillet, and cook for another 2-3 minutes, stirring occasionally.

   - Stir in chopped fresh spinach leaves and cook until wilted, about 1-2 minutes. Add salt and pepper to taste

2. Warm the whole wheat tortillas in the microwave or on a skillet for a few seconds to make them more pliable.

   - Divide the spinach and black bean filling evenly among the tortillas, placing it in the center of each tortilla.

   - Sprinkle shredded reduced-fat cheese over the filling on each tortilla.

3. To roll each burrito, fold the sides of the tortilla over the filling, then fold the bottom edge up and over the filling, tucking it under the filling as you roll tightly.

   - Place the rolled burrito seam side down on a plate or baking sheet.

4. If desired, you can lightly toast the assembled burritos on a skillet or in the oven for a few minutes to crisp up the tortillas.

   - Serve with your choice of toppings, such as salsa, sliced avocado, Greek yogurt, or fresh cilantro.

Notes

• Feel free to add more vegetables to the filling for added flavor and nutrition. Bell peppers, tomatoes, corn, or diced zucchini are great options.

• Adjust the amount of chili powder and smoked paprika to suit your taste preferences. For added spice, you can also add a small pinch of cayenne pepper.

• For more minerals and fiber, choose whole wheat tortillas. If necessary, you can also select gluten-free or low-carb tortillas.

• To prevent the burritos from becoming soggy, you can lightly toast the tortillas before adding the filling. This helps create a barrier and keeps the moisture from the filling from seeping into the tortilla.

• You can prepare the filling in advance and store it in the refrigerator for up to 2-3 days. When ready to serve, simply reheat the filling and assemble the burritos.

• These burritos can be frozen for future meals. Wrap each burrito individually in foil or plastic wrap, then place them in a freezer bag. To reheat, thaw overnight in the refrigerator and then heat in the microwave or oven until warmed through.

Nutritional Information

- Per serving (1 burrito): Calories: 300 kcal, Carbohydrates: 36g, Protein: 15g, Fat: 11g, Saturated Fat: 3g, Cholesterol: 15mg, Sodium: 550mg, Fiber: 9g, Sugar: 2g

SALAD RECIPES

Keto Cobb Salad

Prep Time: 15 minutes
Cook Time: 10 minutes
Servings: 4

For the Salad:
- 6 cups mixed salad greens (lettuce, spinach, arugula)
- 4 hard-boiled eggs, peeled and sliced
- 1 avocado, diced
- 1 cup cooked chicken breast, diced
- 4 slices cooked bacon, crumbled
- 1/2 cup cherry tomatoes, halved
- 1/4 cup crumbled blue cheese
- Salt and pepper to taste

For the Dressing:
- 1/4 cup extra virgin olive oil
- 2 tablespoons apple cider vinegar
- 1 teaspoon Dijon mustard
- 1 clove garlic, minced
- Salt and pepper to taste

Procedure
1. Wash and dry the mixed salad greens and divide them among four serving plates.
   - Slice the hard-boiled eggs and dice the avocado and cooked chicken breast.
   - Crumble the cooked bacon and halve the cherry tomatoes.
   - Arrange the sliced eggs, diced avocado, diced chicken breast, crumbled bacon, and halved cherry tomatoes on top of the mixed salad greens.

2. In a small bowl, whisk together extra virgin olive oil, apple cider vinegar, Dijon mustard, minced garlic, salt, and pepper until well combined. Adjust seasoning to taste.

3. Drizzle the prepared dressing over the assembled salad ingredients.
   - Sprinkle crumbled blue cheese on top of each salad.
   - Season with salt and pepper to taste.

Notes

• Opt for organic, pasture-raised eggs and chicken breast, as well as nitrate-free bacon to ensure the highest quality and healthiest salad possible.

• Feel free to customize the salad with your favorite low-carb vegetables, such as cucumber, bell peppers, or red onion. You can also swap out the blue cheese for another low-carb cheese like feta or goat cheese.

• This salad can be prepped ahead of time for quick and easy meals throughout the week. Store the salad ingredients and dressing separately in airtight containers in the refrigerator, then assemble the salads when ready to eat.

• For added texture, consider adding some toasted nuts or seeds to the salad, such as sliced almonds or pumpkin seeds.

• Enhance the flavor of the salad by adding fresh herbs like parsley or cilantro, or a sprinkle of dried herbs like oregano or thyme to the dressing.

Nutritional Information (per serving)
- Calories: 420 kcal
- Carbohydrates: 9g
- Net Carbs: 5g
- Protein: 24g
- Fat: 32g
- Fiber: 4g
- Sugars: 2g

Tuna Nicoise Salad

Prep Time: 20 minutes
Cook Time: 10 minutes
Servings 4

For the Salad:
- 1 lb small red potatoes, halved
- 4 large eggs
- 8 oz green beans, trimmed
- 4 cups mixed salad greens (lettuce, spinach, arugula)
- 2 (5 oz) cans of tuna, drained
- 1/2 cup cherry tomatoes, halved
- 1/4 cup sliced black olives
- 2 tablespoons capers, drained
- Salt and pepper to taste

For the Dressing:
- 1/4 cup extra virgin olive oil
- 2 tablespoons red wine vinegar
- 1 teaspoon Dijon mustard
- 1 clove garlic, minced
- Salt and pepper to taste

Procedure

1. Place the halved red potatoes in a medium saucepan and cover with water. Bring to a boil, then reduce heat to medium-low and simmer for 10-15 minutes, or until potatoes are fork-tender. Drain and set aside to cool.

   - Meanwhile, place the eggs in a separate saucepan and cover with water. Bring to a boil, then remove from heat, cover, and let eggs sit in hot water for 10-12 minutes. Transfer eggs to a bowl of ice water to cool, then peel and quarter them.

   - Bring a pot of salted water to a boil and blanch the green beans for 2-3 minutes until crisp-tender. To halt the cooking process, drain and immediately transfer to a dish of icy water. Repeatedly drain and pat dry.

2. In a small bowl, whisk together extra virgin olive oil, red wine vinegar, Dijon mustard, minced garlic, salt, and pepper until well combined. Adjust seasoning to taste.

3. Arrange the mixed salad greens on a large serving platter.
  - Top the greens with cooked red potatoes, quartered eggs, blanched green beans, canned tuna, cherry tomatoes, sliced black olives, and capers.
  - Drizzle the prepared dressing over the salad, then season with salt and pepper to taste.

Notes

• Opt for sustainably sourced tuna packed in water or olive oil for the best flavor and texture. Look for fresh, vibrant vegetables and use organic ingredients whenever possible.

• Enhance the flavor of the salad by adding ingredients like thinly sliced red onions, chopped fresh herbs (such as parsley or basil), or anchovy filets. These additions can add depth and complexity to the salad.

• You can omit ingredients like olives or capers if you're not a fan, or add extras like roasted bell peppers or artichoke hearts for additional flavor.

• This salad can be prepared in advance and stored in the refrigerator until ready to serve. Keep the components separate and assemble the salad just before serving to prevent wilting greens or soggy potatoes.

• For a heartier meal, serve with slices of crusty whole grain bread or a side of whole grain crackers. This adds a satisfying crunch and complements the flavors of the salad.

• Any leftover can be stored in an airtight container in the refrigerator for up to 2 days. Enjoy it cold straight from the fridge or let it come to room temperature before serving.

Nutritional Information (per serving)
- Calories: 380 kcal
- Carbohydrates: 25g
- Protein: 25g
- Fat: 20g
- Fiber: 5g
- Sugars: 4g

Cauliflower Potato Salad

Prep Time: 15 minutes
Cook Time: 15 minutes
Servings: 6

Ingredients
- One medium cauliflower head, divided into tiny florets
- 4 hard-boiled eggs, peeled and diced
- 2 stalks celery, finely chopped
- 1/4 cup diced red onion
- 2 tablespoons chopped fresh parsley
- 1/2 cup mayonnaise (use light or sugar-free mayonnaise for a lower calorie option)
- 2 tablespoons Dijon mustard
- 1 tablespoon apple cider vinegar
- 1 teaspoon garlic powder
- Salt and pepper to taste
- Optional: chopped chives for garnish

Procedure
1. Wash the cauliflower head thoroughly and remove the leaves. Cut the cauliflower into small florets, similar in size to traditional potato salad pieces.

2. Heat up a big saucepan of water until it boils. When the cauliflower florets are soft but firm (al dente), add them and simmer for another five to seven minutes. To halt the cooking process, drain the cauliflower and give it a quick rinse under cold water.Dry off with a paper towel or clean kitchen towel

3. In a large mixing bowl, combine the cooked cauliflower, diced hard-boiled eggs, chopped celery, diced red onion, and chopped fresh parsley.

4. In a small bowl, whisk together the mayonnaise, Dijon mustard, apple cider vinegar, garlic powder, salt, and pepper until well combined.

5. Pour the dressing over the cauliflower mixture and gently toss until everything is evenly coated in the dressing.
   - Cover the bowl with plastic wrap or a lid and refrigerate the cauliflower potato salad for at least 1 hour before serving to allow the flavors to meld together.

6. Before serving, garnish the cauliflower potato salad with chopped chives for added freshness and flavor, if desired.
   - Serve chilled as a side dish or light meal option.

Notes

• For extra texture, consider adding chopped pickles or pickle relish to the salad. The crunchy texture will complement the creamy cauliflower and add a burst of flavor.

• Boost the flavor of the salad by adding ingredients like chopped green onions, diced bell peppers, or a sprinkle of paprika. These additions will add depth and complexity to the dish.

• If you prefer a creamier texture, you can increase the amount of mayonnaise or add a dollop of Greek yogurt to the dressing mixture. This will give the salad a richer taste and texture without adding extra carbs.

• You can add herbs like dill, thyme, or basil for a fresh flavor, or a pinch of cayenne pepper for a hint of heat.

• Cauliflower Potato Salad pairs well with grilled chicken, fish, or tofu for a complete and balanced meal. Serve it alongside your favorite protein for a satisfying and nutritious dish.

• Store any leftovers in an airtight container in the refrigerator for up to 3 days. Enjoy the salad cold straight from the fridge or let it come to room temperature before serving.

Nutritional Information (per serving)
- Calories: 150 kcal
- Carbohydrates: 5g
- Protein: 6g
- Fat: 11g
- Fiber: 2g
- Sugars: 2g

Creamy Pesto Chicken Salad with Greens

Prep Time: 15 minutes
Cook Time: 15 minutes
Servings: 4

For the Chicken:
- 1 lb boneless, skinless chicken breasts
- Salt and pepper to taste
- 1 tablespoon olive oil

For the Creamy Pesto Dressing:
- 1/4 cup mayonnaise (use light or sugar-free mayonnaise for a lower calorie option)
- 2 tablespoons prepared pesto sauce
- 1 tablespoon lemon juice
- 1 clove garlic, minced
- Salt and pepper to taste

For the Salad:
- Six cups of mixed greens for salad (arugula, spinach, and lettuce)
- 1/2 cup cherry tomatoes, halved
- 1/4 cup sliced red onion
- 1/4 cup chopped walnuts (optional)
- Grated Parmesan cheese for garnish

Procedure

1. On both sides, season the chicken breasts with salt and pepper. In a skillet over medium heat, warm the olive oil. When the chicken breasts are fully cooked and no longer pink in the center, add the seasoning and cook for 6–7 minutes on each side. Take off the heat and let it cool a little.

2. In a small bowl, whisk together mayonnaise, pesto sauce, lemon juice, minced garlic, salt, and pepper until smooth and well combined. Adjust seasoning to taste.

3. In a large mixing bowl, toss the mixed salad greens with cherry tomatoes, sliced red onion, and chopped walnuts (if using).

4. Slice the cooked chicken breasts into thin strips.

5. Add the sliced chicken to the bowl of salad greens.
   - Pour the creamy pesto dressing over the salad mixture and toss gently until everything is evenly coated in the dressing.

6. Garnish with grated Parmesan cheese and additional chopped walnuts, if desired.
   - Serve immediately as a main dish or light meal option.

<u>Notes</u>
• Feel free to add additional ingredients to the salad to suit your taste preferences. You can include sliced cucumbers, diced bell peppers, or avocado for extra flavor and nutrients.

• This salad can be prepared ahead of time for quick and easy meals throughout the week. Simply store the dressed salad in an airtight container in the refrigerator, and add the sliced chicken just before serving to maintain its freshness.

• If you have leftover cooked chicken from a previous meal, you can use it in this salad to save time. Simply shred or slice the leftover chicken and toss it with the salad greens and dressing.

• If you prefer a more generously dressed salad, you can double the amount of creamy pesto dressing. This will ensure that every bite is coated in delicious flavor.

• For added texture, consider topping the salad with toasted pine nuts or sunflower seeds. The crunchy nuts/seeds will add a satisfying crunch to each bite.

• To make the meal more filling, serve the Creamy Pesto Chicken Salad with a side of whole grain bread or crackers. This will add some carbohydrates to the meal without significantly increasing the overall carb content.

Nutritional Information (per serving)
- Calories: 350 kcal

- Carbohydrates: 5g
- Protein: 25g
- Fat: 25g
- Fiber: 2g
- Sugars: 2g

Cold Asparagus Tomato Salad with Feta

Prep Time: 10 minutes
Cook Time: 5 minutes
Chill Time: 30 minutes
Servings: 4

Ingredients
- 1 lb asparagus, tough ends trimmed
- 1 cup cherry tomatoes, halved
- 1/4 cup crumbled feta cheese
- 2 tablespoons extra virgin olive oil
- 1 tablespoon balsamic vinegar
- 1 clove garlic, minced
- Salt and pepper to taste
- Fresh basil leaves for garnish (optional)

Procedure
1. Boil salted water in a large pot. Add the trimmed asparagus spears and cook for 2-3 minutes, or until they are crisp-tender. Avoid overcooking to maintain their vibrant green color and crisp texture.

   - Once cooked, immediately transfer the asparagus to a bowl of ice water to stop the cooking process. This will help the asparagus retain its bright green color and crispness.After the asparagus has cooled, drain and use paper towels to pat dry.

2. Combine the extra virgin olive oil, balsamic vinegar, minced garlic, salt, and pepper in a small bowl and whisk until thoroughly blended. Taste and adjust the seasoning.

3. Arrange the blanched asparagus spears on a serving platter or individual plates.
   - Scatter the halved cherry tomatoes over the asparagus.
   - Make sure all the salad's ingredients are uniformly coated by pouring the prepared dressing over it.

4. Sprinkle the crumbled feta cheese over the salad, distributing it evenly.

5.   Cover the salad with plastic wrap or a lid and refrigerate for at least 30 minutes to allow the flavors to meld together and the salad to chill.
   - Before serving, garnish with fresh basil leaves if desired.

• For added flavor, consider adding ingredients like chopped fresh herbs such as basil, parsley, or mint to the salad. These herbs will complement the other ingredients and add freshness to the dish.

• To intensify the flavor of the feta cheese, consider toasting it lightly before adding it to the salad. Simply heat a dry skillet over medium heat, add the crumbled feta, and cook for 1-2 minutes, stirring occasionally, until the feta is lightly browned and aromatic.

• To make the salad more filling, you can add protein-rich ingredients such as grilled chicken breast, shrimp, or tofu. Simply grill or cook the protein of your choice separately and add it to the assembled salad before serving.

• If you prefer a vegan version of this salad, you can omit the feta cheese or replace it with a vegan cheese alternative. You can also use a vegan-friendly balsamic vinaigrette dressing instead of the traditional dressing.

• Serve the Cold Asparagus Tomato Salad with Feta alongside slices of crusty whole grain bread or whole wheat pita for a complete and satisfying meal.

• Any leftovers can be kept in the fridge for up to two days if they are kept in an airtight container. Store any leftovers in an airtight container in the refrigerator for up to 2 days.

Nutritional Information (per serving)
- Calories: 110 kcal
- Carbohydrates: 6g
- Protein: 4g
- Fat: 8g

- Fiber: 2g
- Sugars: 3g

Beet and Fonio Salad with Spicy Pickled Carrot

Prep Time: 20 minutes
Cook Time: 15 minutes
Servings: 4

For the Salad:
- 1 cup fonio (or substitute quinoa or couscous)
- 2 medium beets, cooked, peeled, and diced
- 1/4 cup chopped fresh parsley
- 1/4 cup chopped fresh cilantro
- 1/4 cup chopped green onions
- 1/4 cup crumbled feta cheese (optional)
- Salt and pepper to taste

For the spicy pickled carrot
- 1 large carrot, julienned
- 1/4 cup apple cider vinegar
- 1 tablespoon honey or maple syrup (optional for sweetness)
- 1 teaspoon red pepper flakes (adjust to taste)
- 1/2 teaspoon salt

For the Dressing:
- 2 tablespoons extra virgin olive oil
- 1 tablespoon lemon juice
- 1 teaspoon Dijon mustard
- 1 clove garlic, minced
- Salt and pepper to taste

Procedure

1.   In a small saucepan, combine the apple cider vinegar, honey or maple syrup (if using), red pepper flakes, and salt. Bring the mixture to a simmer over medium heat, stirring until the salt and sweetener are dissolved.

   - Add the julienned carrot to the saucepan and cook for 1-2 minutes, just until slightly softened but still crisp.

   - Remove the saucepan from heat and let the pickled carrot cool to room temperature. Once cooled, transfer the pickled carrot and liquid to a glass jar or container. Refrigerate until ready to use.

2.   Two cups of water should be brought to a boil in a medium saucepan. Lower the heat to low and add the rinsed fonio. Once the water has been absorbed and the fonio is soft, simmer it for five minutes.
- After turning off the heat, take the saucepan off of the heat and cover the fonio for five more minutes. Using a fork, fluff the fonio and allow it to come to room temperature.

3.   In a large mixing bowl, combine the cooked and diced beets, chopped parsley, chopped cilantro, chopped green onions, and crumbled feta cheese (if using). Season with salt and pepper to taste.

4. In a small bowl, whisk together the extra virgin olive oil, lemon juice, Dijon mustard, minced garlic, salt, and pepper until well combined.

5.   Add the cooled fonio to the bowl of salad ingredients.
   - Pour the prepared dressing over the salad mixture and toss gently until everything is evenly coated in the dressing.

<u>Notes</u>
• For added depth of flavor, consider roasting the beets instead of boiling them. Simply wrap each beet individually in aluminum foil and roast in a preheated oven at 400°F (200°C) for about 45-60 minutes, or until tender. Before peeling and dicing, allow it to cool.

• If fonio is not available, you can substitute it with cooked quinoa or couscous. Prepare the quinoa or couscous according to package instructions before adding it to the salad.

• Feel free to adjust the amount of red pepper flakes in the pickled carrot to suit your taste preferences. You can lessen or even leave out the red pepper flakes if you'd rather have a softer taste.

• This salad can be prepared ahead of time and stored in the refrigerator until ready to serve. However, it's best to add the dressing and pickled carrot just before serving to maintain the freshness and crunchiness of the ingredients.

• To make this salad a complete meal, you can add protein-rich ingredients such as grilled chicken, tofu, or chickpeas. Simply grill or cook the protein of your choice separately and add it to the assembled salad before serving.

• For additional texture and flavor, consider garnishing the salad with toasted nuts or seeds such as almonds, walnuts, or pumpkin seeds. The crunchy nuts will add a satisfying crunch to each bite.

Nutritional Information (per serving)
- Calories: 200 kcal
- Carbohydrates: 26g
- Protein: 4g
- Fat: 8g
- Fiber: 4g
- Sugars: 5g

DESSERT RECIPES

Frozen Yogurt Pops

Prep Time: 10 minutes
Freezing Time: 4 hours
Servings: 6

Ingredients
- 2 cups Greek yogurt (unsweetened)
- One cup of mixed berries including raspberries, blueberries and strawberries
- Two tablespoons of maple syrup or honey (optional; taste and adjust)

- 1 teaspoon vanilla extract

Procedure
1. In a mixing bowl, combine the Greek yogurt, honey or maple syrup (if using), and vanilla extract. Stir until well combined. Taste and adjust sweetness as desired.

2. Wash and dry the mixed berries. If using strawberries, remove the stems and chop into small pieces. Leave the other berries whole or halve them if they are large.

3. Spoon a small amount of the yogurt mixture into each popsicle mold, filling each about one-third full.
   - Add a few pieces of mixed berries into each mold, distributing them evenly.
   - Continue layering with more yogurt mixture and berries until the molds are almost full. A tiny opening should be left at the top to accommodate expansion during freezing.

4. Place the popsicle sticks into the center of each mold, ensuring they are upright and straight.

5. Carefully transfer the popsicle molds to the freezer and freeze for at least 4 hours, or until completely frozen solid.

6. Once the pops are frozen, remove the molds from the freezer.
   - To unmold the pops, run the bottom of the molds under warm water for a few seconds to loosen them. Gently pull the popsicle sticks to release the pops from the molds.

7. Serve immediately or store them in an airtight container in the freezer until ready to enjoy.

Notes

• Silicone popsicle molds are flexible and make it easier to remove the popsicles once they're frozen. If you don't have silicone molds, you can use traditional popsicle molds or even small paper cups with popsicle sticks inserted into them.

• Get creative with the layering by alternating between different flavors of yogurt and fruits. For example, you can use vanilla yogurt with sliced bananas or mango yogurt with diced pineapple.

• For added texture and crunch, consider mixing in some granola, chopped nuts, or shredded coconut into the yogurt mixture before pouring it into the molds. This will add a delicious contrast to the creamy yogurt and juicy berries.

• Adjust the sweetness of the popsicles to your preference by adding more or less honey or maple syrup. Keep in mind that the sweetness of the berries will also contribute to the overall sweetness of the popsicles.

• For an extra special treat, dip the frozen yogurt pops in melted dark chocolate and sprinkle with chopped nuts or shredded coconut before refreezing. This adds a decadent touch and makes the popsicles feel even more indulgent.

• You can make a batch of Frozen Yogurt Pops ahead of time and keep them in the freezer for up to a month. This way, you'll always have a healthy and refreshing snack on hand whenever you need a sweet treat.

Nutritional Information (per serving)

- Calories: 80 kcal
- Carbohydrates: 10g
- Protein: 6g
- Fat: 1g
- Fiber: 1g
- Sugars: 8g

Dark Chocolate Dipped Cherries

Prep Time: 15 minutes
Cook Time: 5 minutes
Servings: 20

Ingredients
- 1 cup fresh cherries, pitted
- 3 ounces dark chocolate (70% cocoa or higher), chopped
- 1 teaspoon coconut oil
- Sea salt flakes, shredded coconut, or chopped nuts are optional toppings

Procedure
1. Wash the cherries thoroughly under cold water and pat them dry with a paper towel. Use a cherry pitter or a small knife to remove the pits from each cherry. Set aside on a plate lined with parchment paper.

2. Place the chopped dark chocolate and coconut oil in a heatproof bowl. You can use a double boiler or microwave to melt the chocolate. If using a double boiler, place the bowl over a pot of simmering water, making sure the bottom of the bowl doesn't touch the water. Stir the chocolate and coconut oil occasionally until melted and smooth. If using a microwave, heat the chocolate and coconut oil in short bursts of 20-30 seconds, stirring in between, until melted and smooth.

3. Holding each cherry by the stem, dip it into the melted chocolate, swirling to coat evenly. Allow any excess chocolate to drip off before placing the dipped cherry back onto the parchment-lined plate. Repeat with the remaining cherries.

4. If desired, sprinkle the dipped cherries with chopped nuts, shredded coconut, or a pinch of sea salt flakes while the chocolate is still wet. This adds extra flavor and texture to the chocolate-dipped cherries.

5.   Once all the cherries are dipped and decorated, place the plate in the refrigerator for about 10-15 minutes, or until the chocolate has hardened.

6.   Once the chocolate is set, remove the plate from the refrigerator and transfer to a serving platter or airtight container. Serve immediately as a delicious and indulgent treat.

<u>Notes</u>
• Select premium dark chocolate that contains at least 70% cocoa. Dark chocolate contains less sugar than milk chocolate and is rich in antioxidants, making it a better choice for individuals with type 2 diabetes.

• Select ripe, firm cherries for the best flavor and texture. If fresh cherries are not in season, you can use frozen cherries that have been thawed and patted dry with a paper towel.

• To ensure a smooth and glossy finish on the chocolate-dipped cherries, you can temper the chocolate before dipping. Tempering involves melting and cooling the chocolate to specific temperatures to stabilize the cocoa butter crystals. While optional, tempering can help prevent the chocolate from becoming dull or streaky as it sets.

• If you prefer a thicker layer of chocolate on your cherries, you can double dip them after the first layer of chocolate has set. Simply repeat the dipping process once the initial layer of chocolate has hardened, then allow the second layer to set before serving.

• Get creative with the toppings for your chocolate-dipped cherries. In addition to chopped nuts, shredded coconut, or sea salt flakes, you can also try sprinkling them with cocoa powder, crushed freeze-dried fruit, or even a drizzle of melted white chocolate for added visual appeal and flavor.

• Store any leftover chocolate-dipped cherries in an airtight container in the refrigerator for up to 3-4 days. For the best flavor and texture, let them cool to room temperature before serving.

Nutritional Information (per serving, approximately 2 chocolate-dipped cherries)
- Calories: 80 kcal
- Carbohydrates: 10g
- Protein: 1g
- Fat: 5g
- Fiber: 2g
- Sugars: 6g

Lime-Coconut Cream Pie Jars

Prep Time: 20 minutes
Cook Time: 10 minutes
Chilling Time: 4 hours
Servings: Makes 4-6 jars

For the Crust:
- 1 cup almond flour
- 2 tablespoons coconut oil, melted
- 1 tablespoon honey or maple syrup
- 1/2 teaspoon vanilla extract
- Pinch of salt

For the Lime-Coconut Filling:
- 1 can (14 ounces) full-fat coconut milk
- 1/4 cup freshly squeezed lime juice
- Zest of 1 lime
- 1/4 cup honey or maple syrup
- 2 tablespoons cornstarch
- 1/4 cup unsweetened shredded coconut

For Garnish:
- Lime slices
- Toasted shredded coconut

Procedure

1. In a mixing bowl, combine the almond flour, melted coconut oil, honey or maple syrup, vanilla extract, and a pinch of salt. Stir until well combined and the mixture resembles coarse crumbs.

2. Spoon a layer of the almond flour mixture into the bottom of each serving jar, pressing down gently to form a crust. Set aside.

3. In a saucepan, whisk together the coconut milk, lime juice, lime zest, honey or maple syrup, and cornstarch until smooth. While stirring continuously, place the saucepan over medium heat and bring the mixture to a simmer. Cook for 2-3 minutes, or until the mixture thickens.

4. Remove the saucepan from the heat and stir in the shredded coconut until well combined.

5. Pour the filling evenly into each serving jar, covering the almond flour crust. Using a spoon or spatula, level the top surface

6. Place the jars in the refrigerator to chill for at least 4 hours, or until the filling is set and firm.

7. Before serving, garnish each with a slice of lime and a sprinkle of toasted shredded coconut.

Notes

• For the creamiest and most flavorful filling, be sure to use full-fat coconut milk. The higher fat content will help the filling set properly and add richness to the dessert.

• Taste the lime-coconut filling before pouring it into the jars and adjust the sweetness to your preference. If you prefer a sweeter dessert, you can add more honey or maple syrup. Conversely, if you prefer a tangier flavor, you can reduce the amount of sweetener.

• Toasting the shredded coconut before garnishing the jars adds an extra layer of flavor and texture. Simply spread the shredded coconut in a single layer on a baking sheet and bake in a preheated oven at 325°F (160°C) for 5-7 minutes, stirring occasionally, until golden brown and fragrant. Keep a close eye on the coconut to prevent burning.

• These Lime-Coconut Cream Pie Jars can be made ahead of time and stored in the refrigerator for up to 2-3 days. Simply cover the jars with lids or plastic wrap to keep them fresh until ready to serve.

• You can Also add additional flavors or toppings. You can stir in a handful of chopped nuts or chocolate chips into the lime-coconut filling for added crunch, or top the jars with fresh berries or a dollop of whipped coconut cream for a decadent finish.

Nutritional Information (per serving, based on 6 servings)
- Calories: 280 kcal
- Carbohydrates: 20g
- Protein: 4g
- Fat: 22g
- Fiber: 3g
- Sugars: 13g

Lighter Chocolate Cinnamon Pudding

Prep Time: 10 minutes
Cook Time: 10 minutes
Chilling Time: 2 hours
Servings: 4 servings

Ingredients
- 2 cups unsweetened almond milk
- 1/4 cup cornstarch
- 1/4 cup unsweetened cocoa powder
- 1/4 cup honey or maple syrup
- 1 teaspoon vanilla extract
- 1/2 teaspoon ground cinnamon
- Pinch of salt

Procedure

1. In a small bowl, whisk together the cornstarch, cocoa powder, ground cinnamon, and a pinch of salt until well combined. Set aside.

2. In a medium saucepan, heat the unsweetened almond milk over medium heat until it begins to simmer. Stir occasionally to prevent scorching.

3. Once the almond milk is simmering, stir in the honey or maple syrup and vanilla extract until fully dissolved.

4. Gradually sprinkle the dry ingredient mixture into the saucepan with the heated almond milk, whisking continuously to prevent lumps from forming. Cook the pudding mixture for 5-7 minutes, or until it thickens to a smooth and creamy consistency, similar to pudding.

5. Remove the saucepan from the heat and let the pudding cool for a few minutes. Then, transfer the pudding to individual serving cups or ramekins. Cover each cup with plastic wrap, making sure the wrap touches the surface of the pudding to prevent a skin from forming. Chill the pudding in the refrigerator for at least 2 hours, or until set.

6. Once the pudding is chilled and set, remove the plastic wrap and serve the Lighter Chocolate Cinnamon Pudding cold. If preferred, garnish with a dollop of whipped cream or a sprinkle of ground cinnamon.

Notes
• Use high-quality unsweetened cocoa powder and almond milk for the best flavor and texture. Look for almond milk that is unsweetened and fortified with calcium and vitamin D.

• Taste the pudding mixture before chilling and adjust the sweetness to your preference. If you prefer a sweeter pudding, you can add more honey or maple syrup. Alternatively, if you prefer less sweetness, you can reduce the amount of sweetener used.

• Whisk the pudding mixture continuously while cooking to prevent lumps from forming and ensure a smooth and creamy texture. Pay attention to the edges of the saucepan to prevent the pudding from sticking or burning.

• Feel free to customize the pudding by adding additional flavors or toppings. You can stir in a handful of chopped nuts or dark chocolate chips for added texture and flavor, or top each serving with fresh berries or a sprinkle of cocoa powder for a decorative touch.

• Leftover pudding can be stored in an airtight container in the refrigerator for up to 3-4 days. Simply cover the container with a lid or plastic wrap to keep the pudding fresh until ready to enjoy.

• For the best taste and texture, be sure to chill the pudding in the refrigerator for at least 2 hours before serving. Chilled pudding will have a firmer consistency and a refreshing coolness that enhances the overall experience.

Nutritional Information (per serving)
- Calories: 120 kcal
- Carbohydrates: 24g
- Protein: 2g
- Fat: 2g
- Fiber: 2g
- Sugars: 14g

Lemon Basil Custard Pie with Red Berries

Prep Time: 20 minutes
Cook Time: 45 minutes
Chilling Time: 2 hours
Servings: 8

For the Crust:
- 1 1/2 cups almond flour
- 1/4 cup coconut oil, melted
- 2 tablespoons honey or maple syrup
- Pinch of salt

For the Custard Filling:

- 1 cup unsweetened almond milk
- 1/2 cup fresh lemon juice
- Zest of 1 lemon
- 1/2 cup honey or maple syrup
- 4 large eggs
- 2 tablespoons cornstarch
- 1/4 cup fresh basil leaves, finely chopped

For the Topping:
- 1 cup mixed red berries (such as strawberries, raspberries, and/or red currants)
- Fresh basil leaves, for garnish

Procedure

1. Preheat your oven to 350°F (175°C). In a mixing bowl, combine the almond flour, melted coconut oil, honey or maple syrup, and a pinch of salt. Stir until well combined and the mixture resembles coarse crumbs.

- Press the mixture evenly into the bottom and up the sides of a 9-inch pie dish to form the crust. Bake the crust in the preheated oven for 10-12 minutes, or until lightly golden brown. Remove from the oven and let cool while you prepare the filling.

2. In a saucepan, heat the almond milk, lemon juice, lemon zest, and honey or maple syrup over medium heat until it begins to simmer. Whisk the eggs and cornstarch until smooth in another bowl.

- Gradually pour the hot almond milk mixture into the egg mixture, whisking constantly to temper the eggs. Return the mixture to the saucepan and cook over medium heat, stirring constantly, until it thickens to the consistency of custard, about 5-7 minutes.

- Remove the custard from the heat and stir in the finely chopped basil leaves until well combined. Pour the custard filling into the prepared pie crust, spreading it out evenly.

3. To stop a skin from forming, cover the pie with plastic wrap, making sure the wrap contacts the custard's surface. Refrigerate the pie for at least 2 hours, or until the custard is set and chilled.

4. Just before serving, arrange the mixed red berries on top of the chilled pie. Garnish with fresh basil leaves for an extra pop of color and flavor.

<u>Notes</u>

• Taste the custard filling before pouring it into the crust and adjust the sweetness to your preference. If you prefer a sweeter pie, you can add more honey or maple syrup. Conversely, if you prefer a tangier flavor, you can reduce the amount of sweetener used.

• For an extra smooth texture, you can strain the custard mixture through a fine-mesh sieve before pouring it into the pie crust. This will help remove any lumps or bits of cooked egg for a silky-smooth custard.

• Fresh basil leaves add a bright and aromatic flavor to the custard filling. Be sure to use fresh basil rather than dried for the best taste and texture.

• Get creative with the arrangement of the red berries on top of the pie. You can arrange them in a decorative pattern or scatter them randomly for a more rustic look. Feel free to mix and match different types of berries for a variety of colors and flavors.

Nutritional Information (per serving)
- Calories: 280 kcal
- Carbohydrates: 25g
- Protein: 6g
- Fat: 18g
- Fiber: 3g
- Sugars: 18g

Blueberry Ricotta Tart

Prep Time: 20 minutes
Cook Time: 30 minutes
Chilling Time: 1 hour
Servings: 8

For the Crust:
- 1 1/2 cups almond flour

- 1/4 cup coconut oil, melted
- 2 tablespoons honey or maple syrup
- Pinch of salt

For the Filling:
- 1 cup part-skim ricotta cheese
- 1/4 cup plain Greek yogurt
- 2 tablespoons honey or maple syrup
- 1 teaspoon vanilla extract
- Zest of 1 lemon
- 1 large egg
- 1 tablespoon almond flour

For the Topping:
- 1 1/2 cups fresh blueberries
- 1 tablespoon honey or maple syrup
- Fresh mint leaves for garnish (optional)

Procedure

1. Preheat your oven to 350°F (175°C) and lightly grease a 9-inch tart pan with a removable bottom.

   - In a mixing bowl, combine the almond flour, melted coconut oil, honey or maple syrup, and a pinch of salt. Stir until well combined and the mixture resembles coarse crumbs.

   - Press the mixture evenly into the bottom and up the sides of the tart pan to form the crust. Use the back of a spoon or your fingers to press the mixture firmly into place.

   - Preheat the oven and bake the crust for 10 to 12 minutes, or until it begins to become a light golden brown. Take out of the oven and allow it to cool down while you make the filling.

2. In a medium bowl, combine the ricotta cheese, Greek yogurt, honey or maple syrup, vanilla extract, lemon zest, egg, and almond flour. Mix until smooth and well combined.

   - Pour the filling mixture into the cooled tart crust, spreading it out evenly with a spatula.

3. In a small saucepan, heat the blueberries and honey or maple syrup over medium heat. Cook, stirring occasionally, for 5-7 minutes, or until the blueberries start to burst and release their juices.
   - Spoon the cooked blueberries evenly over the ricotta filling in the tart crust.

4. Refrigerate the assembled tart for at least 1 hour, or until the filling is set and chilled.

5. Just before serving, garnish the tart with fresh mint leaves for a pop of color and extra freshness.

Notes

• To ensure a crisp crust, you can blind bake the tart crust before adding the filling. Simply line the tart crust with parchment paper or aluminum foil and fill it with pie weights or dried beans. Bake for 10-12 minutes, then remove the weights and parchment and bake for an additional 5 minutes until lightly golden brown.

• Feel free to customize the tart by using different berries or fruits for the topping. Raspberries, strawberries, or mixed berries would work well in place of blueberries. You can also add a sprinkle of toasted nuts or coconut flakes on top for added texture and flavor.

• This tart can be made ahead of time and stored in the refrigerator for up to 2 days before serving. It's a great option for entertaining or special occasions when you want to prepare dessert in advance.

• For an extra indulgent touch, serve slices of the tart with a dollop of whipped cream or Greek yogurt on top. The creamy topping complements the tartness of the berries and adds a luxurious finish to the dessert.

• Taste the filling and the blueberry topping before assembling the tart and adjust the sweetness according to your preference. If you prefer a sweeter tart, you can add more honey or maple syrup to the filling and topping mixture.

Nutritional Information (per serving)
- Calories: 230 kcal
- Carbohydrates: 18g
- Protein: 7g
- Fat: 16g
- Fiber: 3g

- Sugars: 12g

Sugar-Free Lemon Drizzle Cake

Prep Time: 15 minutes
Cook Time: 40 minutes
Servings: 10

For the Cake:
- 1 1/2 cups almond flour
- 1/2 cup coconut flour
- 1/4 cup granulated sweetener (erythritol, stevia, or monk fruit)
- 1 teaspoon baking powder
- 1/2 teaspoon baking soda
- 1/4 teaspoon salt
- 1/2 cup unsweetened applesauce
- 1/4 cup melted coconut oil
- 3 large eggs
- Zest and juice of 2 lemons
- 1 teaspoon vanilla extract

For the Lemon Drizzle:
- Juice of 1 lemon
- 2 tablespoons powdered sweetener (erythritol, stevia, or monk fruit)

Procedure

1. Preheat your oven to 350°F (175°C) and grease a 9x5-inch loaf pan with coconut oil or line it with parchment paper.

2. In a large mixing bowl, whisk together the almond flour, coconut flour, granulated sweetener, baking powder, baking soda, and salt until well combined.

3.   In a separate bowl, mix together the unsweetened applesauce, melted coconut oil, eggs, lemon zest, lemon juice, and vanilla extract until smooth and well combined.

4. Mix only till blended when combining the wet and dry ingredients. Overmixing may cause the texture to become rough or dense.

5.   Transfer the batter to the prepared loaf pan and spread it out evenly with a spatula. To eliminate any air bubbles, lightly tap the pan against the counter.
 - A toothpick placed into the center of the cake should come out clean after 35 to 40 minutes of baking in a preheated oven.

6. While the cake is baking, prepare the lemon drizzle by mixing together the lemon juice and powdered sweetener until smooth.

7. Once the cake is baked, remove it from the oven and let it cool in the pan for 10 minutes.
   - Use a toothpick or skewer to poke holes all over the top of the cake, then pour the lemon drizzle evenly over the warm cake, allowing it to soak in.

8.   Allow the cake to cool completely in the pan before slicing and serving. Optionally, garnish with additional lemon zest or slices.

<u>Notes</u>
• Choose a granulated sweetener that suits your taste preferences and dietary needs. Erythritol, stevia, and monk fruit sweetener are all popular options for sugar-free baking. To suit your taste, change the amount of sweetener

• Almond flour adds moisture and nutty flavor to the cake. For the greatest texture, use almond flour that has been finely ground.If you prefer a lighter texture, you can sift the almond flour before adding it to the batter.

• When combining the wet and dry ingredients, mix until just combined. Overmixing can result in a dense or tough texture. Use a gentle folding motion to incorporate the ingredients without overworking the batter.

• Keep an eye on the cake as it bakes, as baking times may vary depending on your oven. When a toothpick put into the center comes out clean, the cake is done. A dry cake might be the consequence of overbaking.

• Allow the cake to cool in the pan for 10 minutes before adding the lemon drizzle. Drizzling the lemon syrup over the warm cake allows it to soak in and infuse the cake with extra lemon flavor.

• Store any leftovers in an airtight container at room temperature for up to 3 days, or in the refrigerator for up to 5 days. Another option for extending cake storage is to freeze it. Before serving, let it thaw in the refrigerator

Nutritional Information (per serving)
- Calories: 210 kcal
- Carbohydrates: 8g
- Protein: 6g
- Fat: 16g
- Fiber: 4g
- Sugars: 1g

Keto Peanut Butter Cookies

Prep Time: 10 minutes
Cook Time: 12 minutes
Servings: 12

Ingredients
- 1 cup natural peanut butter (unsweetened)
- 1/3 cup granulated sweetener (erythritol, stevia, or monk fruit)
- 1 large egg
- 1 teaspoon vanilla extract
- Pinch of salt
Optional toppings include chopped nuts or sugar-free chocolate chips

Procedure
1. Line a baking sheet with parchment paper and preheat your oven to 350°F (175°C)

2. In a mixing bowl, combine the natural peanut butter, granulated sweetener, egg, vanilla extract, and a pinch of salt. Stir until all the ingredients are well combined and a dough forms. The dough ought to be somewhat sticky and thick.

3. Using a spoon or cookie scoop, portion out the dough and roll it into balls about 1 inch in diameter. Leaving some space between each cookie, place the balls onto the baking sheet that has been prepared. Gently press down on each cookie with a fork to make a crosshatch design.

4. Transfer the baking sheet to the preheated oven and bake the cookies for 10-12 minutes, or until the edges are lightly golden brown. The cookies will still be soft when they come out of the oven, but they will firm up as they cool.

5. Allow the cookies to cool on the baking sheet for 5 minutes, then transfer them to a wire rack to cool completely. If desired, you can press a few sugar-free chocolate chips or chopped nuts into the tops of the cookies while they are still warm.

6. Any leftovers can be kept for up to five days at room temperature in an airtight container.

Notes
• Choose natural peanut butter that is free of hydrogenated oils and additional sugars. You can use creamy or crunchy peanut butter, depending on your preference. Be sure to stir the peanut butter well before measuring it for the recipe.

• Select a granulated sweetener that suits your taste preferences and dietary needs. Erythritol, stevia, and monk fruit sweetener are all popular options for keto baking.

• Customize the cookies by adding sugar-free chocolate chips, chopped nuts, or a sprinkle of sea salt on top before baking. You can also mix in some cocoa powder for a chocolate twist.

• Keep an eye on the cookies as they bake, as baking times may vary depending on your oven and the size of the cookies. When the edges of the cookies start to become a light golden brown, it's done. They will still be soft when they come out of the oven but will firm up as they cool.

Nutritional Information (per serving - 1 cookie)
- Calories: 120 kcal
- Carbohydrates: 4g

- Protein: 5g
- Fat: 10g
- Fiber: 2g
- Sugars: 1g

VEGETABLE AND SIDES RECIPES

Kale Salad with Creamy Poppy Seed Dressing

Prep Time: 15 minutes
Cook Time: 0 minutes
Servings: 4 servings

For the Salad:
- 1 bunch kale, stems removed and leaves thinly sliced
- 1/4 cup dried cranberries
- 1/4 cup chopped pecans or walnuts
- ¼ cup of goat or feta cheese, crumbled
- 1/4 cup thinly sliced red onion
- 1/4 cup plain Greek yogurt
- 2 tablespoons mayonnaise (use light or low-fat for a lighter option)
- 1 tablespoon apple cider vinegar
- One tablespoon of maple syrup or honey (optional; taste and adjust)
- 1 tablespoon poppy seeds
- Salt and pepper to taste

Procedure

1. Wash the kale thoroughly under cold water and pat it dry with paper towels or a clean kitchen towel. Remove the tough stems and discard them. Stack the kale leaves and thinly slice them into ribbons.

2. In a large mixing bowl, combine the sliced kale, dried cranberries, chopped pecans or walnuts, crumbled feta or goat cheese, and thinly sliced red onion. Mix the ingredients until they are all spread equally.

3. In a small bowl, whisk together the plain Greek yogurt, mayonnaise, apple cider vinegar, honey or maple syrup (if using), and poppy seeds until smooth and creamy. Season the dressing with salt and pepper to taste.

4. Pour the creamy poppy seed dressing over the kale salad, starting with half of the dressing initially. Mix the ingredients until they are all spread equally. Add more dressing as needed, depending on your preference for creaminess.

5. Optionally, garnish with additional dried cranberries, chopped nuts, or crumbled cheese on top for extra flavor and visual appeal.

Notes

• Before assembling the salad, consider massaging the kale leaves with a bit of olive oil and lemon juice. This helps to tenderize the kale and reduce its bitterness, making it more enjoyable to eat.

2. You can add ingredients like sliced almonds, pumpkin seeds, sunflower seeds, or dried cherries for variation.

3. You can prepare the salad ingredients and dressing ahead of time and store them separately in the refrigerator. When ready to serve, toss the salad with the dressing just before serving to maintain its freshness and crispness.

4. If you prefer a sweeter dressing, you can increase the amount of honey or maple syrup in the dressing. Conversely, if you prefer a tangier dressing, you can add a bit more apple cider vinegar.

5. To turn this salad into a complete meal, consider adding a source of lean protein such as grilled chicken, salmon, tofu, or chickpeas on top. This will add satiety and make the salad more filling.

6. For a dairy-free option, you can omit the cheese or use a dairy-free alternative such as vegan feta or nutritional yeast.

Nutritional Information (per serving)
- Calories: 180 kcal
- Carbohydrates: 18g
- Protein: 6g
- Fat: 10g
- Fiber: 3g
- Sugars: 10g

Roasted Garlic-Parmesan Cabbage

Prep Time: 10 minutes
Cook Time: 25 minutes
Servings: 4 servings

Ingredients
- 1 medium head of cabbage
- 2 tablespoons olive oil
- 4 cloves garlic, minced
- 2 tablespoons grated Parmesan cheese
- Salt and pepper to taste
- Fresh parsley, chopped (for garnish, optional)

Procedure
1. Preheat your oven to 400°F (200°C). Line a baking sheet with parchment paper or lightly grease it with olive oil.

2. Remove any outer leaves from the cabbage and rinse it under cold water. Cut the cabbage into wedges, leaving the core intact to hold the leaves together.

3. In a small skillet, heat 1 tablespoon of olive oil over medium heat. Add the minced garlic and sauté for 1-2 minutes, or until fragrant. Remove from heat and set aside.

4. Place the cabbage wedges on the prepared baking sheet. Drizzle the remaining olive oil over the cabbage wedges and use your hands to evenly coat them with oil. Sprinkle the minced garlic over the cabbage, making sure to distribute it evenly. Season the cabbage with salt and pepper to taste.

5. Transfer the baking sheet to the preheated oven and roast the cabbage for 20-25 minutes, or until the edges are golden brown and crispy, and the cabbage is tender when pierced with a fork.

6. Remove the roasted cabbage from the oven and sprinkle the grated Parmesan cheese over the top of each wedge. Return the baking sheet to the oven and roast for an additional 2-3 minutes, or until the cheese is melted and lightly golden.

7. Garnish with chopped fresh parsley, if desired, for a pop of color and freshness.

Notes
• You can add other herbs and spices such as thyme, rosemary, or red pepper flakes for extra flavor.

• Keep an eye on the cabbage while it's roasting to prevent it from burning. The edges should turn golden brown and crispy, while the cabbage should be tender when pierced with a fork.

• For the best flavor, use freshly grated Parmesan cheese rather than pre-grated cheese. It will melt beautifully and add a rich, nutty flavor to the roasted cabbage.

• Consider serving the roasted cabbage with a side of marinara sauce or aioli for dipping. The tanginess of the sauce complements the savory flavors of the cabbage and Parmesan cheese.

• To make this recipe vegan, simply omit the Parmesan cheese or use a dairy-free alternative such as nutritional yeast or vegan Parmesan.

• If you have leftovers, you can use them to make a delicious stir-fry or add them to soups and stews for extra flavor and texture.

Nutritional Information (per serving):
- Calories: 110 kcal
- Carbohydrates: 10g
- Protein: 3g
- Fat: 7g
- Fiber: 5g
- Sugars: 4g

Curried Cauliflower with Mint Yogurt Sauce

Prep Time: 15 minutes
Cook Time: 25 minutes
Servings: 4 servings

For the Curried Cauliflower:
- 1 large head cauliflower, cut into florets
- 2 tablespoons olive oil
- 2 teaspoons curry powder
- 1 teaspoon ground cumin
- 1 teaspoon ground coriander
- 1/2 teaspoon turmeric powder
- Salt and pepper to taste

For the Mint Yogurt Sauce:
- 1/2 cup plain Greek yogurt
- 1/4 cup chopped fresh mint leaves
- 1 tablespoon lemon juice
- Salt and pepper to taste

Procedure

1. Preheat your oven to 425°F (220°C). Cut the cauliflower into florets and place them in a large mixing bowl. Pour on some olive oil and toss to ensure even coating

2. In a small bowl, combine the curry powder, cumin, coriander, turmeric, salt, and pepper. Sprinkle the spice mixture over the cauliflower florets and toss until they are evenly coated.

3. Spread the seasoned cauliflower florets in a single layer on a baking sheet lined with parchment paper. Roast in the preheated oven for 20-25 minutes, or until the cauliflower is tender and golden brown, stirring halfway through the cooking time for even browning.

5. While the cauliflower is roasting, prepare the mint yogurt sauce. In a small bowl, combine the Greek yogurt, chopped fresh mint leaves, lemon juice, salt, and pepper. Stir until well combined. Adjust the seasoning to taste.

6. Drizzle the mint yogurt sauce over the roasted cauliflower or serve it on the side as a dipping sauce.

Notes

• If you prefer a milder flavor, reduce the amount of curry powder, or omit it altogether. Conversely, if you enjoy spicy food, you can add a pinch of cayenne pepper or red chili flakes to the spice mixture.

• Fresh mint leaves add a refreshing flavor to the yogurt sauce. If you don't have fresh mint on hand, you can use dried mint instead, but the flavor may be less vibrant. Alternatively, you can substitute fresh cilantro or parsley for a different herbaceous twist.

• Curried cauliflower pairs well with whole grains like brown rice, quinoa, or couscous. Serve the roasted cauliflower over a bed of cooked grains for a more substantial meal that's rich in fiber and nutrients.

• To make this dish a complete meal, consider adding a protein source such as grilled chicken, chickpeas, or tofu. Simply toss the protein with the cauliflower and spices before roasting, or serve it on the side for a balanced meal

• For added texture and flavor, sprinkle the roasted cauliflower with chopped nuts like almonds or pistachios before serving. The nuts add a satisfying crunch and a dose of healthy fats to the dish.

Nutritional Information (per serving)
- Calories: 120 kcal
- Carbohydrates: 10g
- Protein: 6g
- Fat: 7g
- Fiber: 4g
- Sugars: 5g

Air-Fryer Beets with Feta

Prep Time: 10 minutes
Cook Time: 25 minutes
Servings: 4 servings

Ingredients

- 4 medium-sized beets, peeled and sliced into 1/4-inch rounds
- 1 tablespoon olive oil
- 1 teaspoon dried thyme
- Salt and pepper to taste
- 1/4 cup crumbled feta cheese
- Fresh parsley, chopped, for garnish (optional)

Procedure

1. For around five minutes, preheat your air fryer to 375°F (190°C). Peel the beets and slice them into rounds about 1/4 inch thick. Place the beet slices in a large bowl.

2. Drizzle the olive oil over the beet slices and sprinkle with dried thyme, salt, and pepper. Toss the beets until they are evenly coated with the seasonings.

3. Arrange the seasoned beet slices in a single layer in the air fryer basket. You may need to cook the beets in batches depending on the size of your air fryer. Cook the beets at 375°F (190°C) for about 20-25 minutes, flipping them halfway through the cooking time, until they are tender and slightly crispy on the edges.

4. Sprinkle the crumbled feta cheese over the top of the beets. Garnish with chopped fresh parsley if desired. They pair well with grilled meats, roasted vegetables, or a simple green salad.

Notes

• Look for firm, smooth-skinned beets with vibrant color when selecting them at the grocery store. Fresh beets will yield the best flavor and texture in this recipe.

• Try to slice the beets into uniform rounds so that they cook evenly in the air fryer. This ensures that all the beets are cooked to the same degree of doneness.

• You can experiment with different herbs and spices such as rosemary, thyme, garlic powder, or smoked paprika to enhance the flavor of the beets.

• If you prefer sweeter beets, you can drizzle them with a touch of honey or maple syrup before air-frying. This adds a subtle sweetness that complements the earthy flavor of the beets.

• If you're not a fan of feta cheese, you can substitute it with crumbled goat cheese or blue cheese for a tangy flavor twist.

• They make a great addition to salads, grain bowls, or charcuterie boards.

Nutritional Information (per serving):
- Calories: 90 kcal
- Carbohydrates: 8g
- Protein: 3g
- Fat: 5g
- Fiber: 2g
- Sugars: 6g

Strawberry Spinach Salad with Buttermilk Dressing

Prep Time: 15 minutes
Cook Time: 0 minutes
Servings: 4 servings

For the salad:
- 6 cups fresh baby spinach leaves
- 1 cup sliced fresh strawberries
- 1/4 cup sliced almonds, toasted
- 2 tablespoons crumbled feta cheese (optional)

- 2 tablespoons thinly sliced red onion (optional)

For the dressing:
- 1/4 cup low-fat buttermilk
- 2 tablespoons plain Greek yogurt
- 1 tablespoon extra-virgin olive oil
- 1 tablespoon honey
- 1 tablespoon apple cider vinegar
- 1 teaspoon Dijon mustard
- Salt and pepper to taste

Procedure

1. Wash the baby spinach leaves thoroughly and pat them dry with a clean kitchen towel or salad spinner. Slice the strawberries into thin slices. If using, toast the sliced almonds in a dry skillet over medium heat until lightly golden and fragrant. Crumble the feta cheese and thinly slice the red onion.

2. Toss the baby spinach leaves, sliced strawberries, toasted almonds, crumbled feta cheese, and sliced red onion (if using) into a large salad dish. Toss gently to mix everything together evenly.

3. In a small bowl, whisk together the buttermilk, Greek yogurt, olive oil, honey, apple cider vinegar, Dijon mustard, salt, and pepper until smooth and well combined. Adjust the seasoning to taste, adding more salt and pepper if needed.

4. Drizzle the prepared buttermilk dressing over the salad ingredients in the bowl. Start with a small amount of dressing and toss the salad gently to coat the ingredients evenly. Don't overdress the salad; only add more dressing as needed.

5. Garnish with additional sliced strawberries, almonds, and crumbled feta cheese if desired.

6. Pair it with grilled chicken or fish for a complete meal.

Notes
• For optimal flavor, choose strawberries that are ripe and fresh. If strawberries are not in season, you can substitute with other seasonal fruits like raspberries, blueberries, or sliced peaches.

• Toasting the almonds enhances their nutty flavor and adds crunch to the salad. Be careful not to over-toast them as they can burn quickly. Keep an eye on them and stir frequently while toasting.

• The buttermilk dressing can be prepared ahead of time and stored in an airtight container in the refrigerator for up to 3 days. Give it a good shake or stir before using it on the salad.

4. You can add avocado slices, cucumber slices, or even cooked quinoa for extra texture and flavor.

• For the best taste and texture, serve the salad chilled. You can chill the salad bowl in the refrigerator before assembling the ingredients to keep the salad crisp and refreshing.

• To prevent the salad from becoming soggy, dress it with the buttermilk dressing just before serving. This helps to maintain the crispness of the spinach leaves and freshness of the strawberries.

Nutritional Information (per serving)
- Calories: 150 kcal
- Carbohydrates: 15g
- Protein: 5g
- Fat: 8g
- Fiber: 4g
- Sugars: 8g

Roasted Carrots and Parsnips

Prep Time: 10 minutes
Cook Time: 30 minutes
Servings: 4 servings

Ingredients

- 4 medium carrots, peeled and cut into sticks
- Cut four medium parsnips into sticks after peeling them.
- 2 tablespoons olive oil
- 1 teaspoon dried thyme
- Salt and pepper to taste
- Fresh parsley, chopped, for garnish (optional)

Procedure

1. Set an oven temperature of 400°F (200°C) and cover a baking sheet with aluminum foil or parchment paper.

2. Peel the carrots and parsnips, then cut them into sticks approximately 2-3 inches long and 1/2 inch thick. Place them in a large bowl.

3. Drizzle the olive oil over the carrots and parsnips, then sprinkle with dried thyme, salt, and pepper. Once the oil and seasonings are equally distributed over the veggies, toss them

4. Spread the seasoned carrots and parsnips in a single layer on the prepared baking sheet. guarantee uniform cooking, make sure they are not crowded.

5. Place the baking sheet in the preheated oven and roast the vegetables for about 25-30 minutes, or until they are tender and lightly caramelized, ensure even browning, stir halfway through the cooking process.

6. Garnish with freshly chopped parsley if desired.

<u>Notew</u>

• Try to cut the carrots and parsnips into uniform sticks to ensure they cook evenly. This helps to avoid some pieces becoming overcooked while others remain undercooked.

• While dried thyme works well in this recipe, you can also use fresh herbs like rosemary or sage for added flavor. Simply chop the herbs finely and toss them with the vegetables before roasting.

• If you prefer sweeter roasted vegetables, you can drizzle them with a little honey or maple syrup before roasting. This adds a touch of sweetness that complements the natural sweetness of the carrots and parsnips.

• Make sure the carrots and parsnips are spread out in a single layer on the baking sheet. Overcrowding the pan can cause the vegetables to steam rather than roast, resulting in a less crispy texture.

• Keep an eye on the vegetables towards the end of the cooking time to prevent them from burning. They should be tender when pierced with a fork and lightly caramelized on the edges.

• For an extra flavor boost, serve the roasted carrots and parsnips with a dipping sauce or aioli. A simple garlic aioli or balsamic glaze pairs beautifully with the earthy flavors of the vegetables.

Nutritional Information (per serving):
- Calories: 120 kcal
- Carbohydrates: 18g
- Protein: 2g
- Fat: 5g
- Fiber: 6g
- Sugars: 6g

Brussels Sprouts with Bacon, Garlic & Shallots

Prep Time: 10 minutes
Cook Time: 25 minutes
Servings: 4 servings

Ingredients
- 1 lb Brussels sprouts, trimmed and halved
- 4 slices bacon, chopped
- 2 shallots, thinly sliced
- 3 cloves garlic, minced
- 2 tablespoons olive oil
- Salt and pepper to taste

Procedure

1. Preheat your oven to 400°F (200°C). Cut the Brussels sprouts in half lengthwise after trimming the ends. After giving them a quick rinse in cold water, use paper towels to pat dry.

2. In a large oven-safe skillet or cast-iron pan, cook the chopped bacon over medium heat until it becomes crispy and browned. Remove the cooked bacon from the pan and set it aside on a plate lined with paper towels to drain excess grease.

3. In the same skillet with the bacon drippings, add the sliced shallots and minced garlic. Sauté them for 2-3 minutes, or until they become fragrant and translucent.

4. Add the halved Brussels sprouts to the skillet with the shallots and garlic. Add a drizzle of olive oil and taste-test salt and pepper for seasoning. Toss everything together until the Brussels sprouts are evenly coated in the bacon drippings and oil.

5. Transfer the skillet to the preheated oven and roast the Brussels sprouts for 20-25 minutes, or until they are tender and caramelized, stirring halfway through the cooking time for even browning.

6. Once the Brussels sprouts are roasted to your desired level of crispiness, remove the skillet from the oven. Sprinkle the crispy bacon pieces over the roasted Brussels sprouts and gently toss to combine.

<u>**Notes**</u>

• Make sure to cut the ends of the Brussels sprouts and remove any outer leaves that are yellowed or damaged before halving them. This ensures that they cook evenly and have a nice appearance.

• For extra crispy bacon, you can bake it in the oven separately while the Brussels sprouts are roasting. Place the bacon slices on a baking sheet lined with parchment paper and bake at 400°F (200°C) for 15-20 minutes, or until crispy. This method reduces the amount of grease in the dish and allows the bacon to cook more evenly.

• You can add other ingredients like diced apple, dried cranberries, or chopped nuts for added flavor and texture.

• You can prepare the Brussels sprouts, bacon, shallots, and garlic ahead of time and store them separately in the refrigerator. When ready to serve, simply assemble the dish and roast the Brussels sprouts in the oven.

• If you have any leftovers, you can use them to make delicious Brussels sprouts and bacon frittata, or add them to salads, grain bowls, or pasta dishes for added flavor and nutrients.

Nutritional Information (per serving):
- Calories: 180 kcal
- Carbohydrates: 12g
- Protein: 7g
- Fat: 13g
- Fiber: 4g

- Sugars: 3g

FISH AND SEAFOOD RECIPES

Cracker Crusted Cod

Prep Time: 10 minutes
Cook Time: 15 minutes
Servings: 4

Ingredients
- 4 cod filets about 6 ounce each
- 1 cup whole grain crackers, crushed into fine crumbs
- 2 tablespoons grated Parmesan cheese
- 1 teaspoon dried parsley
- 1/2 teaspoon garlic powder
- 1/2 teaspoon paprika
- Salt and pepper to taste
- 2 tablespoons olive oil
- Lemon wedges for serving

Procedure
1. Preheat your oven to 400°F (200°C). To make cleanup easier, line a baking sheet with parchment paper.

2. In a shallow dish, combine the crushed whole grain crackers, grated Parmesan cheese, dried parsley, garlic powder, paprika, salt, and pepper. To uniformly mix all the ingredients, give it a good stir.

3. Use paper towels to pat the cod filets dry. Mix well to combine all the ingredients evenly.

3. Pat the cod filets dry with paper towels. Brush each filet with olive oil on both sides.

4. Press each cod filet into the cracker crumb mixture, ensuring that the filets are evenly coated on both sides. Press the cracker mixture onto the fish to help it adhere.

5. Transfer the coated cod filets to the baking sheet that has been ready. Drizzle a little extra olive oil over the top of each filet for added moisture and crispiness.

6. Place the baking sheet in the preheated oven and bake the cod filets for 12-15 minutes, or until the fish is opaque and flakes easily with a fork. The cracker crust should be golden brown and crispy.

7. Serve hot with lemon wedges on the side for squeezing over the fish.Serve the cracker crusted cod with a side of steamed vegetables or a green salad for a complete meal.

Nutritional Information (per serving)
Calories: 250 kcal
Protein: 25g
Fat: 10
Carbohydrates: 15g
 Fiber: 2g

Pistachio Crusted Halibut

Prep Time: 15 minutes
Cook Time: 15 minutes
Servings: 4

Ingredients
- 4 halibut filets (about 6 ounces each)
- 1 cup shelled pistachios, finely chopped
- 2 tablespoons olive oil
- 2 tablespoons Dijon mustard
- 2 tablespoons honey or maple syrup

- 1 tablespoon lemon juice
- 1 teaspoon garlic powder
- Salt and pepper to taste
- Lemon wedges for serving
- Fresh parsley for garnish (optional)

Procedure

1. Preheat your oven to 400°F (200°C). make cleanup easier, line a baking sheet with parchment paper.

2. In a shallow dish, combine the finely chopped pistachios with garlic powder, salt, and pepper. Stir to mix well.

3. In a separate bowl, whisk together the olive oil, Dijon mustard, honey or maple syrup, and lemon juice until well combined. Pat the halibut filets dry with paper towels, then brush both sides of each filet with the mustard mixture.

4. Press each mustard-coated halibut filet into the pistachio mixture, ensuring that the filet is evenly coated on both sides with the pistachio crust. Gently press the pistachios onto the fish to help them adhere.

5. Place the pistachio-crusted halibut filets on the prepared baking sheet. Fish should be baked for 12 to 15 minutes in a preheated oven, or until it is opaque and flakes readily with a fork. Crispy and golden brown is how the crust should look.

6. Serve with a side of steamed vegetables or a green salad for a complete meal.

Nutritional Information (per serving)
Calories: 350 kcal
Protein: 30g
Fat: 20g
Carbohydrates: 12g
Fiber: 3g

Grilled Shrimp Skewers with Creamy Chili Sauce

Prep Time: 20 minutes
Cook Time: 10 minutes
Servings: 4

For the Shrimp Skewers:
- 1 pound large shrimp, peeled and deveined
- 2 tablespoons olive oil
- 2 cloves garlic, minced
- 1 teaspoon smoked paprika
- 1/2 teaspoon ground cumin
- Salt and pepper to taste
- Lemon wedges for serving

For the Creamy Chili Sauce:
- 1/2 cup plain Greek yogurt
- 1 tablespoon mayonnaise
- 1 tablespoon fresh lime juice
- 1 tablespoon chopped cilantro
- 1 teaspoon chili powder
- 1/2 teaspoon garlic powder
- Salt and pepper to taste

Procedure

1. In a bowl, combine the peeled and deveined shrimp with olive oil, minced garlic, smoked paprika, ground cumin, salt, and pepper. Toss until the shrimp are evenly coated with the marinade. Let them marinate for at least 15 minutes in the refrigerator.

2. Preheat your grill to medium-high heat. To avoid burning, submerge wooden skewers in water for at least half an hour.

3. To guarantee consistent cooking, thread the marinated shrimp onto the skewers, leaving a small space between each shrimp.

4. Put the shrimp skewers on the grill that has been prepared. Cook the shrimp for two to three minutes on each side, or until they are opaque, pink, and have grill marks. Take care not to overcook them; if cooked for an extended period of time, shrimp may turn tough.

5. Make the creamy chili sauce while the shrimp are frying. Combine the Greek yogurt, mayonnaise, chopped cilantro, fresh lime juice, garlic powder, chili powder, salt, and pepper in a small bowl. Taste and adjust the seasoning to suit your needs.

6. Serve with creamy chili sauce on the side for dipping. Garnish with fresh cilantro and lemon wedges or you can serve the grilled shrimp skewers with a side of steamed vegetables or a green salad for a complete meal.

Nutritional Information (per serving)
Calories: 200 kcal
Protein: 25g
Fat: 9g
Carbohydrates: 4g
Fiber: 1g

Shrimp Scampi

Prep Time: 10 minutes
Cook Time: 10 minutes
Servings: 4

Ingredients
- One pound medium shrimp deveined and peeled
- 8 ounces linguine or spaghetti
- 4 tablespoons unsalted butter
- 4 cloves garlic, minced
- 1/4 teaspoon red pepper flakes (adjust to taste)
- Zest of 1 lemon
- Juice of 1 lemon

- 1/4 cup dry white wine (optional)
- Salt and pepper to taste
- 2 tablespoons chopped fresh parsley
- Grated Parmesan cheese for serving (optional)

Procedure

1. Cook the linguine or spaghetti according to the package instructions until al dente. Drain the pasta, reserving 1/2 cup of the pasta cooking water, and set aside.

2. Pat the peeled and deveined shrimp dry with paper towels. Add a dash of pepper and salt for seasoning.

3. Melt two tablespoons of butter in a large skillet over medium heat. When the shrimp are pink and opaque, add them to the skillet and cook them for two to three minutes on each side. Take out of the skillet and reserve the cooked shrimp.

4. Melt the last two tablespoons of butter in the same skillet. Add the red pepper flakes and minced garlic, and simmer for one to two minutes, or until aromatic. Take care to prevent the garlic from burning.

5. Add the cooked pasta to the skillet with the garlic butter sauce. Toss to coat the pasta evenly. Use a small amount of the pasta boiling water that was set aside to soften up any dry pasta.

6. Stir in the lemon zest, lemon juice, and dry white wine (if using).Simmer for a further one to two minutes to let the flavors combine.

7. Return the cooked shrimp to the skillet and toss to combine with the pasta and sauce. Cook for an additional minute until the shrimp is heated through. Stir in the chopped fresh parsley.

8. Add salt and pepper to taste. Divide the shrimp scampi pasta among serving plates. If preferred, garnish with more chopped parsley and grated Parmesan cheese.

Nutritional Information (per serving)
Calories: 400 kcal
Protein: 25g
Fat: 12g
Carbohydrates: 45g

Fiber: 2g

Broiled Rainbow Trout with Lemon Oil and Oven-Grilled Vegetable

Prep Time: 15 minutes
Cook Time: 20 minutes
Servings: 4

Ingredients
- Four rainbow trout filets, weighing roughly six ounces each
- 2 tablespoons olive oil
- Zest of 1 lemon
- Juice of 1 lemon
- 2 cloves garlic, minced
- 1 teaspoon dried thyme
- Salt and pepper to taste
- 2 cups mixed vegetables (such as bell peppers, zucchini, and cherry tomatoes), cut into bite-sized pieces
- 1 tablespoon balsamic vinegar
- Fresh parsley for garnish (optional)

Procedure
1. Preheat your oven's broiler on high. Place the oven rack in the top position, about 6 inches from the heat source. To make cleanup easier, line a baking pan with aluminum foil.

2. Use paper towels to pat the rainbow trout filets dry. Put them on the baking sheet that has been prepared, skin side down.

3. In a small bowl, whisk together the olive oil, lemon zest, lemon juice, minced garlic, dried thyme, salt, and pepper. Brush the lemon oil marinade generously over the tops of the trout filets.

4. Place the baking sheet under the preheat broiler and broil the trout filets for 8-10 minutes, or until they are cooked through and the tops are golden brown and slightly crispy. Monitor them to avoid burning

5. While the trout is broiling, spread the mixed vegetables out on another baking sheet. Drizzle with olive oil, balsamic vinegar, salt, and pepper, and toss to coat evenly. Place the baking sheet in the oven underneath the trout and roast for 10-12 minutes, or until the vegetables are tender and lightly charred around the edges.

6. Once the trout and vegetables are cooked, remove them from the oven. Transfer the trout filets to serving plates and divide the oven-grilled vegetables among them. Garnish with fresh parsley if desired.

Nutritional Information (per serving)
- Calories: 250 kcal
- Protein: 25g
- Fat: 12g
- Carbohydrates: 10g
- Fiber: 3g

Garlic Ginger Mackerel

Prep Time: 10 minutes
Cook Time: 15 minutes
Servings: 4

Ingredients
- 4 mackerel filets (about 6 ounces each)
- 4 cloves garlic, minced
- 1 tablespoon grated fresh ginger
- 2 tablespoons low-sodium soy sauce
- 1 tablespoon rice vinegar
- 1 tablespoon honey or maple syrup

- 1 tablespoon olive oil
- Salt and pepper to taste
- Fresh cilantro for garnish (optional)

Procedure

1. In a small bowl, combine the minced garlic, grated ginger, soy sauce, rice vinegar, honey or maple syrup, olive oil, and a pinch of salt and pepper. Stir well to combine. Place the mackerel filets in a shallow dish or resealable plastic bag, and pour the marinade over them. Ensure the filets are evenly coated with the marinade. To give the flavors time to meld, cover the dish or seal the bag and place it in the refrigerator for at least half an hour.

2. Preheat your oven to 400°F (200°C). Line a baking sheet with parchment paper or aluminum foil for easy cleanup.

3. Remove the marinated mackerel filets from the refrigerator and place them on the prepared baking sheet. Discard any excess marinade. Bake the mackerel in the preheated oven for 12-15 minutes, or until the fish is cooked through and flakes easily with a fork. The cooking time may vary depending on the thickness of the filets, so keep an eye on them to avoid overcooking.

4. For an extra burst of flavor, you can garnish the mackerel filets with a squeeze of fresh lime juice and additional minced cilantro before serving.

Nutritional Information (per serving)
Calories: 250 kcal
Protein: 25g
Fat: 15g
Carbohydrates: 5g
Fiber: 0.5g

Salmon Filets with Hot Mango Chutney

Prep Time: 10 minutes
Cook Time: 15 minutes

Ingredients
- 4 salmon filets (about 6 ounces each)
- 1 cup diced mango (fresh or frozen)
- 1/4 cup apple cider vinegar
- 2 tablespoons honey or maple syrup
- 1 tablespoon grated fresh ginger
- 1 teaspoon ground cumin
- 1/2 teaspoon ground coriander
- 1/4 teaspoon red pepper flakes (adjust to taste)
- Salt to taste
- 1 tablespoon olive oil
- Fresh cilantro for garnish (optional)

Procedure
1. In a small saucepan, combine the diced mango, apple cider vinegar, honey or maple syrup, grated ginger, ground cumin, ground coriander, red pepper flakes, and a pinch of salt. Stir well to combine.

2. After setting the saucepan on medium heat, simmer the mixture. Cook for 8-10 minutes, stirring occasionally, until the mango is soft and the mixture has thickened to a chutney-like consistency. Taste and adjust seasoning as needed. Remove from heat and set aside.

3. While the mango chutney is cooking, preheat your oven to 400°F (200°C). Pat the salmon filets dry with paper towels and season both sides with a pinch of salt.

4. In a large oven-safe skillet, heat the olive oil over medium-high heat. When the skillet is hot, place the salmon filets in it, skin side down. Sear for 2-3 minutes until the skin is crispy and golden brown.

5. Transfer the skillet to the preheated oven and bake the salmon filets for 8-10 minutes, or until they are cooked through and flake easily with a fork.

6. For an extra burst of flavor, you can garnish the salmon filets with a squeeze of fresh lime juice and additional red pepper flakes before serving.

Nutritional Information (per serving)
Calories: 350 kcal
Protein: 30g
Fat: 18g
Carbohydrates: 20g
Fiber: 2g

Shellfish Risotto

Prep Time: 15 minutes
Cook Time: 30 minutes
Servings: 4

Ingredients
- 1 cup Arborio rice
- 1/2 cup dry white wine
- Four cups of low-sodium vegetable or chicken broth
- 1 tablespoon olive oil
- 1 small onion, finely chopped
- 2 cloves garlic, minced
- 1/2 pound mixed shellfish (such as shrimp, scallops, and/or mussels), cleaned and deveined
- 1/4 cup grated Parmesan cheese
- 2 tablespoons chopped fresh parsley
- Salt and pepper to taste

Procedure
1. In a medium saucepan, heat the chicken or vegetable broth over low heat. While you make the risotto, keep it warm

2. In a large skillet or Dutch oven, heat the olive oil over medium heat. Cook the finely chopped onion for three to four minutes, or until it becomes transparent. Add the minced garlic and heat until fragrant, about one more minute

3. Add the Arborio rice to the skillet with the onions and garlic. Mix thoroughly to coat the rice with the oil. Toast the rice for 2-3 minutes, stirring constantly, until it becomes translucent around the edges.

4. Pour the dry white wine into the skillet with the rice. Stir continuously until the wine is absorbed by the rice.

5. Ladle one ladleful at a time into the skillet with the heated chicken or veggie broth. Make repeated stirs in the rice and wait for each ladleful of broth to absorb completely before adding more. This process should be repeated until the rice is soft and creamy but still somewhat al dente. 20 to 25 minutes should be needed for this.

6. Prepare the shellfish during the risotto's cooking process. A little olive oil should be heated over medium-high heat in a different skillet. Add the cleaned and deveined shellfish to the skillet and cook until they are opaque and cooked through, about 2-3 minutes for shrimp and scallops, and until the mussels have opened.

7. Once the risotto is cooked to your desired consistency, add the cooked shellfish to the skillet with the risotto. Mix thoroughly and thoroughly warm.

8. Divide the shellfish risotto among serving plates or bowls. Garnish with additional Parmesan cheese and parsley if desired. Serve immediately. For an extra burst of flavor, you can garnish the shellfish risotto with a drizzle of olive oil, a sprinkle of red pepper flakes, or some lemon zest before serving.

Nutritional Information (per serving)
Calories: 350 kcal
Protein: 20g
Fat: 8g
 Carbohydrates: 50g
Fiber: 2g

Cumin-Crusted Fish Fillet with Lemon

Prep Time: 10 minutes

Cook Time: 10 minutes

Servings: 4

Ingredients

- 4 fish filets (such as tilapia, cod, or halibut), about 4-6 ounces each
- 2 teaspoons ground cumin
- 1 teaspoon paprika
- 1/2 teaspoon garlic powder
- 1/2 teaspoon ground coriander
- Salt and pepper to taste
- 2 tablespoons olive oil
- 1 lemon, sliced for serving
- Fresh parsley or cilantro for garnish (optional)

Procedure

1. Preheat your oven to 400°F (200°C). Line a baking sheet with parchment paper or lightly grease it to prevent sticking.

2. Ground cumin, paprika, ground coriander, garlic powder, salt, and pepper should all be combined in a small basin. Toss to blend well.

3. Pat the fish filets dry with paper towels. Sprinkle both sides of each filet evenly with the spice mixture, pressing lightly to adhere the spices to the fish.

4. In a large saucepan, warm up olive oil over medium-high heat. Once hot, add the seasoned fish filets to the skillet, being careful not to overcrowd the pan. Cook for 2-3 minutes on each side, or until the fish is lightly browned and crispy on the outside.

5. Carefully transfer the seared fish filets to the prepared baking sheet. After the oven has been preheated, place the baking sheet inside and bake for a further five to seven minutes, or until the fish is cooked through and flakes easily with a fork.

6. For an extra burst of freshness, you can garnish the cooked fish filets with additional lemon slices or wedges and a sprinkle of fresh parsley or cilantro before serving.

Nutritional Information (per serving)

Calories: 200 kcal

Protein: 25g
Fat: 10g
Carbohydrates: 1g
Fiber: 0.5g

Sole with Parsley and Mint

Prep Time: 15 minutes
Cook Time: 10 minutes
Servings: 4

Ingredients
- 4 sole filets (about 4-6 ounces each)
- 1/4 cup fresh parsley, finely chopped
- 2 tablespoons fresh mint, finely chopped
- 2 tablespoons olive oil
- 2 cloves garlic, minced
- 1 lemon, juiced
- Salt and pepper to taste

Procedure
1. Preheat your oven to 375°F (190°C). Line a baking sheet with parchment paper or lightly grease it to prevent sticking.

2. In a small bowl, combine the finely chopped parsley and mint. Set aside.

3. Pat the sole filets dry with paper towels and place them on the prepared baking sheet. Drizzle each filet with olive oil and minced garlic. Drizzle the filets with freshly squeezed lemon juice and season with salt and pepper to taste.

4. Sprinkle the chopped parsley and mint mixture evenly over the top of each sole filet, pressing lightly to adhere the herbs to the fish.

5. Transfer the baking sheet to the preheated oven and bake the sole filets for 8-10 minutes, or until the fish is cooked through and easily flakes with a fork.

6. For an extra burst of flavor, you can garnish the cooked sole filets with additional lemon slices or wedges and a sprig of fresh parsley or mint before serving.

Nutritional Information (per serving)
Calories: 180 kcal
Protein: 25g
Fat: 8g
Carbohydrates: 1g

Fiber: 0.5g

POULTRY RECIPES

Lemon Herb Roasted Chicken

Prep Time: 10 minutes
Cook Time: 1 hour 30 minutes
Servings: 4 servings

Ingredients
- 1 whole chicken (about 3-4 pounds)
- 2 tablespoons olive oil
- 2 cloves garlic, minced
- 1 lemon, zest and juice
- 1 teaspoon of dried rosemary or 1 tablespoon of fresh rosemary leaves
- 1 tablespoon fresh rosemary leaves (or 1 teaspoon dried rosemary)
- Salt and pepper to taste
- 1 onion, quartered
- 2 carrots, chopped
- 2 celery stalks, chopped
- 1 cup low-sodium chicken broth or water

Procedure
1. Preheat your oven to 375°F (190°C). After giving the chicken a thorough rinse in cold water, blot it dry with paper towels. Transfer the chicken to a sizable baking dish or roasting pan.

2. In a small bowl, mix together the olive oil, minced garlic, lemon zest, lemon juice, thyme, rosemary, salt, and pepper to form a paste.

3. Rub the herb mixture all over the chicken, making sure to coat it evenly, including under the skin if possible. Place the quartered onion, chopped carrots, and chopped celery around the chicken in the roasting pan.

4. Roast the chicken in the preheated oven for about 1 hour 30 minutes, or until the internal temperature reaches 165°F (75°C) when measured with a meat thermometer inserted into the thickest part of the thigh without touching bone.

5. Every 30 minutes, baste the chicken with the pan juices to keep it moist and flavorful. After cooking, take the chicken out of the oven and give it ten to fifteen minutes to rest before slicing. Along with the vegetables and pan juices, serve the roasted chicken

Nutritional Information (per serving)
- Calories: 350 kcal
- Carbohydrates: 6g
- Protein: 30g
- Fat: 22g
- Saturated Fat: 5g
- Cholesterol: 95mg
- Sodium: 320mg
- Fiber: 2g
- Sugars: 2g

Chipotle Cauliflower & Turkey Chili

Prep Time: 15 minutes
Cook Time: 45 minutes
Servings: 6 servings

Ingredients
- 1 tablespoon olive oil
- 1 onion, chopped
- 3 cloves garlic, minced
- 1 pound lean ground turkey
- 1 teaspoon ground cumin
- 1 teaspoon chili powder
- 1 teaspoon smoked paprika
- 1/2 teaspoon dried oregano

- 1/2 teaspoon ground coriander
- 1/4 teaspoon cayenne pepper (optional, for extra heat)
- 1 can (14.5 ounces) diced tomatoes
- One can (15 ounces) of rinsed and drained kidney beans
- One tiny head of cauliflower, divided into tiny florets
- 1 minced chipotle pepper in adobo sauce - 2 cups low-sodium vegetable or chicken broth
- Salt and pepper to taste
Optional toppings: chopped fresh cilantro, diced avocado, Greek yogurt, shredded cheese

Procedure
1. Heat the olive oil in a large pot over medium heat. Add the chopped onion and minced garlic and sauté until softened, about 3-4 minutes.

2. Add the ground turkey to the pot and cook, breaking it up with a spoon, until browned and cooked through, about 5-7 minutes. Stir in the ground cumin, chili powder, smoked paprika, dried oregano, ground coriander, and cayenne pepper (if using). Cook until aromatic, one or two more minutes.

3. Add the diced tomatoes (with their juices), black beans, kidney beans, chopped cauliflower, minced chipotle pepper, and chicken or vegetable broth to the pot. Stir to combine.

4. Bring the chili to a simmer, then reduce the heat to low. Cover and let it simmer for about 30-35 minutes, stirring occasionally, until the cauliflower is tender and the flavors have melded together.

5. Taste the chili and season with salt and pepper as needed, depending on your preference. Ladle the chipotle cauliflower and turkey chili into bowls and serve hot. Optionally, top each serving with chopped fresh cilantro, diced avocado, Greek yogurt, or shredded cheese.

<u>**Notes**</u>
• Adjust the amount of chipotle pepper and cayenne pepper according to your preference for spiciness. If you prefer a milder chili, you can reduce or omit the cayenne pepper and use less chipotle pepper.

• If you prefer a vegetarian version of this chili, you can omit the ground turkey and use extra vegetables or substitute with plant-based protein sources like tofu or tempeh.

Nutritional Information (per serving)
- Calories: 270 kcal
- Carbohydrates: 26g
- Protein: 23g
- Fat: 9g
- Saturated Fat: 2g
- Cholesterol: 35mg
- Sodium: 450mg
- Fiber: 9g
- Sugars: 5g

Orange Chicken Spinach Salad

Prep Time: 15 minutes
Cook Time: 15 minutes
Servings: 4 servings

For the Orange Chicken:
- 1 pound boneless, skinless chicken breasts, cut into bite-sized pieces
- 2 tablespoons olive oil
- Salt and pepper to taste
- 1/2 cup orange juice (freshly squeezed is best)
- 2 tablespoons low-sodium soy sauce
- 1 tablespoon honey or maple syrup
- 2 cloves garlic, minced
- 1 teaspoon grated fresh ginger
- Zest of 1 orange
- 1 tablespoon cornstarch
- 2 tablespoons water

For the Salad:
- 6 cups fresh spinach leaves, washed and dried
- 1 orange, peeled and sliced
- 1/4 cup sliced red onion
- 1/4 cup sliced almonds, toasted
Optional: sliced avocado, crumbled feta cheese

Procedure

1. Add salt and pepper to the chicken pieces for seasoning. A big skillet filled with one tablespoon of olive oil is heated to medium-high heat. After adding the chicken to the skillet, heat it for 6 to 8 minutes, or until it is browned and cooked through. After taking the chicken out of the skillet, set it aside.

2. Add the last tablespoon of olive oil to the same skillet. When aromatic, add the minced garlic and grated ginger and sauté for one to two minutes. Add the orange juice, soy sauce, honey or maple syrup, and orange zest to the skillet. Stir to combine and bring to a simmer.

3. In a small bowl, mix the cornstarch with water until dissolved. Stir thoroughly after adding the cornstarch mixture to the skillet. Simmer for an additional one to two minutes, or until the sauce thickens.

4. Return the cooked chicken to the skillet and toss to coat it in the orange sauce. Allow it to simmer for another 2-3 minutes until heated through.

5. In a large salad bowl, combine the fresh spinach leaves, sliced orange, sliced red onion, and toasted sliced almonds. Toss to combine.

6. Divide the salad among serving plates and top each serving with the orange chicken pieces. Optionally, add sliced avocado and crumbled feta cheese on top.

Notes

• For even more flavor, you can marinate the chicken in a mixture of orange juice, soy sauce, garlic, and ginger for 30 minutes to 1 hour before cooking. This will infuse the chicken with the delicious citrus and savory flavors.

• If you enjoy extra crunch in your salad, you can add additional toasted nuts or seeds, such as pumpkin seeds or sunflower seeds, along with the sliced almonds.

Nutritional Information (per serving)
- Calories: 320 kcal
- Carbohydrates: 21g
- Protein: 27g
- Fat: 15g
- Saturated Fat: 2g
- Cholesterol: 65mg
- Sodium: 450mg
- Fiber: 5g
- Sugars: 11g

Balsamic Butter Chicken Bites

Prep Time: 10 minutes
Cook Time: 15 minutes
Servings: 4 servings

For the Balsamic Butter Sauce:
- 2 tablespoons balsamic vinegar
- 2 tablespoons low-sodium soy sauce
- 1 tablespoon honey or maple syrup
- 2 cloves garlic, minced
- 1 teaspoon grated fresh ginger
- 2 tablespoons unsalted butter
- Salt and pepper to taste

For the Chicken Bites:
- One pound of skinless, boneless chicken breasts, sliced into small pieces
- 2 tablespoons olive oil
- Salt and pepper to taste
- Optional garnish: chopped fresh parsley or green onions

Procedure

1. In a small bowl, whisk together the balsamic vinegar, low-sodium soy sauce, honey or maple syrup, minced garlic, and grated ginger until well combined. Set aside.

2. Add salt and pepper to the chicken pieces for seasoning. Warm up some olive oil in a big skillet over medium high heat. Add the chicken pieces to the skillet and cook until browned and cooked through, about 6-8 minutes, stirring occasionally to ensure even cooking.

3. Once the chicken is cooked, reduce the heat to medium-low and add the balsamic butter sauce to the skillet. Stir well to coat the chicken pieces in the sauce. Allow the sauce to simmer for 2-3 minutes, stirring occasionally, until it thickens slightly and coats the chicken evenly.

4. Once the sauce has thickened and coated the chicken, remove the skillet from the heat. Add salt and pepper. Optionally, garnish with chopped fresh parsley or green onions for added flavor and color.

5. Serve the Balsamic Butter Chicken Bites hot as a delicious main dish or as a protein-packed appetizer. They pair well with a variety of sides such as steamed vegetables, quinoa, or a mixed green salad.

Notes

• If you prefer a thicker sauce, you can mix 1-2 teaspoons of cornstarch with a little water to make a slurry. Stir the slurry into the sauce during the simmering step and continue to cook until the sauce reaches your desired consistency.

• For a complete meal, consider adding some vegetables to the skillet along with the chicken. Bell peppers, mushrooms, and snap peas are all great options that pair well with the flavors of the balsamic butter sauce.

Nutritional Information (per serving)
- Calories: 260 kcal
- Carbohydrates: 8g
- Protein: 27g
- Fat: 13g
- Saturated Fat: 4g
- Cholesterol: 85mg
- Sodium: 400mg
- Fiber: 0.5g

- Sugars: 6g

Lemony Chicken and Rice Soup

Prep Time: 10 minutes
Cook Time: 30 minutes
Servings: 4 servings

Ingredients
- 1 tablespoon olive oil
- 1 onion, diced
- 2 carrots, diced
- 2 celery stalks, diced
- 2 cloves garlic, minced
- 6 cups low-sodium chicken broth
- 1 cup cooked brown rice
- 2 cups cooked chicken breast, shredded or diced
- Zest and juice of 1 lemon
- Salt and pepper to taste
- Fresh parsley, chopped (for garnish)

Procedure
1. In a big pot, warm up the olive oil over medium heat. Add the diced onion, carrots, and celery to the pot and sauté for about five minutes, or until they start to soften. When aromatic, add the minced garlic and simmer for one more minute.

2. Pour in the low-sodium chicken broth and bring the mixture to a boil. Reduce the heat to low and let the soup simmer for 15-20 minutes, allowing the flavors to meld together.

3. Once the vegetables are tender and the soup has simmered, add cooked brown rice and cooked chicken breast to the pot. Stir well to combine and let the soup simmer for another 5-10 minutes to heat through.

4. Stir in the zest and juice of one lemon to brighten up the flavors of the soup. Add salt and pepper.

<u>Notes</u>
• Consider adding other fresh herbs like thyme or dill to the soup for added flavor complexity. You can either add them during the simmering process or sprinkle them on top as a garnish before serving.

• Feel free to customize the soup with other vegetables you have on hand or prefer. Bell peppers, peas, or spinach would all be great additions to this versatile soup.

Nutritional Information (per serving)
- Calories: 250 kcal
- Carbohydrates: 20g
- Protein: 25g
- Fat: 8g
- Saturated Fat: 1.5g
- Cholesterol: 60mg
- Sodium: 400mg
- Fiber: 3g
- Sugars: 4g

Hearty Chicken Gyros

Prep Time: 15 minutes
Cook Time: 20 minutes
Servings: 4 servings

For the Chicken:
- One lb boneless and skinless chicken breasts
- 2 tablespoons olive oil
- 2 cloves garlic, minced
- 1 teaspoon dried oregano
- 1 teaspoon dried thyme

- 1 teaspoon paprika
- Salt and pepper to taste

For the Tzatziki Sauce:
- 1 cup plain Greek yogurt
- Grate and squeeze one cucumber to get rid of extra moisture.
- 2 cloves garlic, minced
- 1 tablespoon fresh lemon juice
- 1 tablespoon fresh dill, chopped
- Salt and pepper to taste

For Serving:
- 4 whole wheat pita breads
- 1 cup cherry tomatoes, halved
- 1/2 red onion, thinly sliced
- 1 cup shredded lettuce
- 1/4 cup crumbled feta cheese (optional)
- Lemon wedges for serving

Procedure

1. In a bowl, combine olive oil, minced garlic, dried oregano, dried thyme, paprika, salt, and pepper. Add the chicken breasts to the marinade, ensuring they are evenly coated. In the fridge, let the chicken marinade for at least half an hour.

2. In another bowl, mix together the Greek yogurt, grated cucumber, minced garlic, lemon juice, chopped dill, salt, and pepper. Stir until well combined. Refrigerate the tzatziki sauce until ready to use.

3. A skillet or grill pan should be heated to medium-high heat. After taking the chicken breasts out of the marinade, put them on the heated skillet. Cook the chicken for 6 to 8 minutes on each side, or until it is thoroughly done and no longer has any pink in the center. Take the chicken off the burner and give it a break for a few minutes before slicing.

4. Warm the whole wheat pita bread either in the microwave or on the grill for a few seconds. Place a generous spoonful of tzatziki sauce on each pita bread. Top with sliced chicken, cherry tomatoes, red onion, shredded lettuce, and crumbled feta cheese if desired.

5. Roll up the filled pita breads and secure them with toothpicks if necessary. Serve with lemon wedges on each side

Notes
• For added flavor and texture, lightly grill the pita bread before assembling the gyros. This step will give the bread a slight char and make it more pliable for wrapping.

• Consider adding a dollop of hummus to each gyro for extra creaminess and flavor. Choose a low-fat or homemade hummus to keep the dish diabetes-friendly.

Nutritional Information (per serving)
- Calories: 350 kcal
- Carbohydrates: 28g
- Protein: 30g
- Fat: 13g
- Saturated Fat: 3g
- Cholesterol: 75mg
- Sodium: 400mg
- Fiber: 5g
- Sugars: 6g

Chicken and Broccoli with Dill Sauce

Prep Time: 15 minutes
Cook Time: 20 minutes
Servings: 4 servings

For the Chicken:
- 1 lb boneless, skinless chicken breasts, thinly sliced
- 2 tablespoons olive oil
- Salt and pepper to taste

For the Broccoli:
- 1 head broccoli, cut into florets

- 2 cloves garlic, minced
- 2 tablespoons olive oil
- Salt and pepper to taste

For the Dill Sauce:
- 1 cup plain Greek yogurt
- 2 tablespoons fresh dill, chopped
- 1 tablespoon lemon juice
- 1 clove garlic, minced
- Salt and pepper to taste

Procedure

1. Season the thinly sliced chicken breasts with salt and pepper. In a big pot, warm up the olive oil over medium heat. Add the seasoned chicken slices to the skillet and cook for about 4-5 minutes on each side, or until cooked through and golden brown. After cooking, take the chicken out of the skillet and place it aside.

2. In the same skillet, add another tablespoon of olive oil and minced garlic. Sauté for about 1 minute until fragrant. Add the broccoli florets to the skillet and season with salt and pepper. Cook, stirring occasionally, for about 5-6 minutes, or until the broccoli is tender but still crisp.

3. In a small bowl, mix together the Greek yogurt, chopped dill, lemon juice, minced garlic, salt, and pepper. Stir until well combined.

4. Arrange the cooked chicken slices and sautéed broccoli on a serving platter. Drizzle the dill sauce over the chicken and broccoli, or serve it on the side as a dipping sauce.

5. Garnish the dish with additional fresh dill if desired. Serve immediately while still warm.

<u>Notes</u>

• If you like a bit of spice, consider adding a pinch of red pepper flakes or a dash of hot sauce to the dill sauce for a kick of heat.

• Feel free to customize the dill sauce by adding other fresh herbs like parsley, chives, or basil for additional flavor complexity.

• For a more balanced meal, serve the chicken and broccoli with whole grains such as brown rice, quinoa, or whole wheat couscous. These complex carbohydrates will provide sustained energy and additional fiber.

Nutritional Information (per serving)
- Calories: 280 kcal
- Carbohydrates: 8g
- Protein: 30g
- Fat: 14g
- Saturated Fat: 2g
- Cholesterol: 75mg
- Sodium: 160mg
- Fiber: 3g
- Sugars: 3g

Chicken-Spaghetti Squash Bake

Prep Time:** 20 minutes
Cook Time:** 1 hour
Servings:** 4 servings

Ingredients
- 1 medium spaghetti squash
- 2 cups cooked chicken breast, shredded
- 1 cup marinara sauce (sugar-free)
- 1 cup shredded mozzarella cheese
- 1/4 cup grated Parmesan cheese
- 1 teaspoon olive oil
- 2 cloves garlic, minced
- 1/2 teaspoon dried oregano
- 1/2 teaspoon dried basil
- Salt and pepper to taste
- Fresh basil leaves for garnish (optional)

Procedure

1. Preheat your oven to 400°F (200°C). Split the spaghetti squash in half lengthwise, then use a spoon to remove the seeds and membranes. Add salt and pepper to the sliced sides after brushing them with olive oil. Spoon the cut side of the squash halves onto a parchment paper-lined baking sheet. Bake for 40 to 45 minutes, or until the squash is soft and pierces easily with a fork, in a preheated oven. Take it out of the oven and let it cool down a little.

2. Once the spaghetti squash is cool enough to handle, use a fork to scrape the flesh into strands. Place the spaghetti squash strands in a large mixing bowl.

3. In a separate pot, warm up olive oil over medium heat. Add minced garlic and sauté until fragrant, about 1 minute. Add the shredded chicken breast to the skillet along with dried oregano and basil. Season with salt and pepper to taste. Cook for 3-4 minutes, stirring occasionally, until the chicken is heated through and well coated with the herbs and garlic.

4. Add the cooked chicken to the bowl with the spaghetti squash strands. Pour marinara sauce over the chicken and squash, and toss gently to combine. Spread the mixture evenly in a baking dish after transferring it there.

5. Sprinkle shredded mozzarella cheese and grated Parmesan cheese evenly over the top of the chicken-spaghetti squash mixture. Place the baking dish in the oven and bake for an additional 15-20 minutes, or until the cheese is melted and bubbly.

6. Once baked, remove the Chicken-Spaghetti Squash Bake from the oven and let it cool for a few minutes. If desired, garnish with fresh basil leaves and serve hot!

<u>Notes</u>

For added flavor and texture, you can incorporate diced vegetables like bell peppers, onions, or mushrooms into the chicken-spaghetti squash mixture before baking. Simply sauté the vegetables along with the garlic until they're tender, then combine them with the chicken and spaghetti squash strands. This not only enhances the nutritional profile of the dish but also adds more color and flavor to the final bake.

Nutritional Information (per serving)
- Calories: 300 kcal
- Carbohydrates: 16g
- Protein: 30g

- Fat: 14g
- Saturated Fat: 6g
- Cholesterol: 80mg
- Sodium: 550mg
- Fiber: 4g
- Sugars: 6g

Turkey Patties with Avocado

Prep Time: 15 minutes
Cook Time: 15 minutes
Servings; 4

Ingredients
- 1 pound lean ground turkey
- 1 ripe avocado, mashed
- 1/4 cup finely chopped onion
- 2 cloves garlic, minced
- 1 teaspoon ground cumin
- 1/2 teaspoon paprika
- 1/4 teaspoon black pepper
- 1/4 teaspoon salt
- 2 tablespoons olive oil

For serving
- Whole grain buns or lettuce leaves (for low-carb option)
- Tomato slices
- Lettuce leaves
- Sliced red onion
- Mustard or your favorite sauce

Procedure

1. In a large mixing bowl, combine the ground turkey, mashed avocado, chopped onion, minced garlic, ground cumin, paprika, black pepper, and salt. Stir thoroughly to ensure that all ingredients are combined equally.

2. Form each of the four equal portions of the ingredients into a patty that is about 1/2 inch thick.

3. In a skillet over medium heat, warm the olive oil. When the skillet is heated, add the turkey patties, being careful not to pack it too full. They might need to be cooked in batches.

4. Cook the patties until they are cooked through and have an internal temperature of 165°F (75°C), about 5 to 6 minutes on each side. The patties should no longer have a pink core and instead have a golden brown outside.

5. While the patties are cooking, prepare your desired toppings and assemble your burgers. You can use whole grain buns or lettuce leaves as the base, then top with tomato slices, lettuce leaves, sliced red onion, and your favorite sauce.

6. Before serving, take the cooked patties out of the skillet and allow them to settle for a few minutes

7. Serve the turkey patties with avocado immediately, along with your chosen toppings. Enjoy your delicious and nutritious meal!

Notes
• You can prepare the turkey patties ahead of time and store them in the refrigerator for up to 24 hours before cooking. This can help save time on busy weeknights.

• While the recipe calls for cooking the patties in a skillet, you can also grill them for a smoky flavor or bake them in the oven for a healthier option.

• Get creative with your burger toppings! Try adding sliced avocado, roasted red peppers, or a dollop of Greek yogurt instead of traditional mayo.

• Pair the turkey patties with a side salad, steamed vegetables, or sweet potato fries for a well-rounded meal.

• You can also freeze the uncooked turkey patties for later use. Simply shape the patties and place them on a baking sheet lined with parchment paper. Freeze until solid, then transfer to a freezer-safe bag or container. Thaw in the refrigerator before cooking.

Nutritional Information (per serving)
- Calories: 280
- Total Fat: 18g
- Saturated Fat: 3g
- Cholesterol: 55mg
- Sodium: 240mg
- Total Carbohydrates: 6g
- Dietary Fiber: 3g
- Sugars: 1g
- Protein: 24g

SOUP AND STEW RECIPES

Cream of Avocado Soup

Prep Time 10 minutes
Cook Time: 10 minutes
Servings: 4

Ingredients:
- 2 ripe avocados
- 1 small onion, chopped
- 2 cloves garlic, minced
- 3 cups low-sodium vegetable broth
- 1/2 cup plain Greek yogurt
- 2 tablespoons lime juice
- 1/4 cup chopped cilantro
- Salt and pepper to taste
- **Optional toppings**: diced tomatoes, sliced green onions, Greek yogurt, or tortilla strips

Procedure:
1. Begin by preparing the avocados. Remove the pits by cutting them in half lengthwise. Remove the flesh with a spoon and transfer it to a food processor or blender.

2. In a medium saucepan, heat a drizzle of olive oil over medium heat. Add the chopped onion and minced garlic. Simmer for about 5 minutes, or until the onion is tender and transparent.

3. Add the cooked onion and garlic mixture to the blender or food processor with the avocado.

4. Pour the vegetable broth into the blender or food processor with the avocado mixture. Blend until smooth and creamy.

5. Transfer the blended mixture back to the saucepan. Warm thoroughly over medium-low heat, stirring from time to time.

6. Once the soup is heated, remove it from the heat. Stir in the Greek yogurt, lime juice, and chopped cilantro. Add salt and pepper to taste.

7. Ladle the soup into bowls and garnish with your desired toppings, such as diced tomatoes, sliced green onions, a dollop of Greek yogurt, or tortilla strips. Serve immediately and enjoy!

Nutritional Information (per serving):
- Calories: 200
- Total Fat: 15g
- Saturated Fat: 2g
- Cholesterol: 2mg
- Sodium: 300mg
- Total Carbohydrates: 12g
- Dietary Fiber: 8g
- Sugars: 2g
- Protein: 6g

Gingery Chicken Soup with Zucchini Noodles

Prep Time: 15 minutes
Cook Time: 25 minutes
Servings: 4

Ingredients
- 1 tablespoon olive oil
- 1 small onion, diced
- 2 cloves garlic, minced
- 1 tablespoon fresh ginger, grated

- 2 medium carrots, peeled and sliced
- 2 stalks celery, sliced
- 4 cups low-sodium chicken broth
- 2 cups cooked chicken breast, shredded
- 2 medium zucchinis, spiralized into noodles
- Salt and pepper to taste
- Fresh cilantro or parsley for garnish (optional)

Procedure

1. In a big pot, warm up the olive oil over medium heat. Add the chopped onion and cook for 3–4 minutes, or until transparent.

2. Cook the grated ginger and minced garlic in the pot for a further minute, or until fragrant.

3. Add sliced carrots and celery to the pot, and cook for 5 minutes until slightly softened.

4. Pour in the chicken broth and bring the soup to a simmer. Cook the vegetables for ten to fifteen minutes, or until they are soft.

5. Stir in the shredded chicken breast and zucchini noodles, and cook for another 5 minutes until the zucchini noodles are just tender.

6. To taste, add salt and pepper to the soup for seasoning

7. Serve the soup hot, garnished with fresh cilantro or parsley if desired.

<u>Notes</u>

• You can customize this soup by adding other vegetables like spinach, bell peppers, or mushrooms for added flavor and nutrients. Just adjust the cooking time accordingly to ensure all vegetables are cooked to your desired level of tenderness.

Nutritional Information
- Calories: Approximately 200 kcal
- Total Fat: 7g
- Saturated Fat: 1g
- Cholesterol: 50mg
- Sodium: 300mg
- Total Carbohydrates: 8g

- Dietary Fiber: 2g
- Sugars: 4g
- Protein: 25g

Barley and Pumpkin Beef Stew

Prep Time: 15 minutes
Cook Time: 1 hour 30 minutes
Servings: 6

Ingredients
- 1 lb (450g) lean beef stew meat, cut into bite-sized pieces
- 1 cup pearl barley, rinsed
- 1 small pumpkin, peeled, seeded, and cubed
- 2 carrots, peeled and diced
- 2 celery stalks, diced
- 1 onion, diced
- 3 cloves garlic, minced
- 4 cups low-sodium beef broth
- 1 cup water
- 1 tablespoon olive oil
- 1 teaspoon dried thyme
- 1 teaspoon dried rosemary
- Salt and pepper to taste
- Fresh parsley, chopped (for garnish)

Procedure
1. Heat olive oil in a large pot over medium heat. Simmer for about 5 minutes, or until the onion is tender and transparent

2. Add the minced garlic and cook for another minute until fragrant.

3. Add the beef stew meat to the pot and brown on all sides, about 5-7 minutes.

4. Once the meat is browned, add the diced carrots, celery, and cubed pumpkin to the pot. Stir well to combine.

5. Pour in the beef broth and water, then add the rinsed pearl barley, dried thyme, dried rosemary, salt, and pepper. Stir to combine all ingredients.

6. After bringing the stew to a boil, turn down the heat. Cover and simmer for about 1 hour, stirring occasionally, until the beef is tender and the barley is cooked through.

7. Once the stew is cooked, taste and adjust seasoning if needed. If the stew is too thick, you can add more water or beef broth to reach your desired consistency.

8. Serve hot, garnished with chopped fresh parsley for a burst of freshness.

Nutritional Information (per serving)
- Calories: 320 kcal
- Protein: 25g
- Carbohydrates: 30g
- Fat: 10g
- Fiber: 7g
- Sugar: 5g
- Sodium: 480mg

Cauliflower Soup with Hazelnuts and Bacon

Prep Time: 15 minutes
Cook Time: 30 minutes
Servings: 4

Ingredients
- 1 large head cauliflower, chopped into florets
- 4 slices bacon, chopped
- 1 onion, diced
- 2 cloves garlic, minced
- 4 cups low-sodium chicken or vegetable broth

- 1/2 cup roasted hazelnuts, chopped
- 1/2 cup heavy cream (optional)
- Salt and pepper to taste
- Fresh parsley, chopped (for garnish)

Procedure

1. In a large pot, cook the chopped bacon over medium heat until crispy. Remove the bacon from the pot and set it aside on a paper towel-lined plate to drain excess fat. One tablespoon or so of bacon fat should remain in the pot.

2. In the same pot with the bacon fat, add the diced onion and minced garlic. Simmer for about 5 minutes, or until the onion is tender and transparent.

3. Add the cauliflower florets to the pot and sauté for another 5 minutes, allowing them to slightly brown.

4. Pour in the chicken or vegetable broth, ensuring that the cauliflower is submerged. Bring the mixture to a boil, then reduce the heat to low and let it simmer for about 15-20 minutes, or until the cauliflower is fork-tender.

5. Puree the soup with an immersion blender until it's smooth. As an alternative, you can transfer the soup to a blender in batches and process it until it's smooth. Be cautious when blending hot liquids.

6. Once the soup is smooth, stir in the heavy cream (if using) to add richness to the soup. To taste, add salt and pepper for seasoning

7. Garnish each serving with the crispy bacon, chopped roasted hazelnuts, and fresh parsley.

Nutritional Information (per serving, without heavy cream)
- Calories: 200 kcal
- Protein: 10g
- Carbohydrates: 15g
- Fat: 12g
- Fiber: 5g
- Sugar: 5g

- Sodium: 400mg

CONCLUSION

As we come to the end of this journey through the world of managing Type 2 Diabetes through diet, let's take a moment to reflect on the key points we've covered and to reinforce the importance of long-term commitment to your health.

Throughout this cookbook, we've explored the fundamental principles of a Type 2 Diabetes diet: low sugar, low carb, and nutrient-dense meals. We've discovered how these dietary choices can help regulate blood sugar levels, improve insulin sensitivity, and promote overall well-being. By embracing a variety of delicious, easy-to-prepare recipes, we've empowered ourselves to take control of our health and enjoy flavorful meals without compromising our dietary goals.

One of the most important lessons we've learned is the significance of balance. Balancing macronutrients—such as carbohydrates, proteins, and fats—allows us to maintain stable blood sugar levels and provides sustained energy throughout the day. By incorporating a diverse range of fruits, vegetables, lean proteins, and healthy fats into our meals, we can create a nutritionally rich diet that supports our body's needs while minimizing the risk of diabetes-related complications.

In addition to balance, consistency is key to long-term success. Consistently making healthy food choices, monitoring portion sizes, and staying physically active are essential habits for managing Type 2 Diabetes effectively. While it may require dedication and effort, the rewards of improved health and well-being are well worth the commitment.

As you embark on your journey beyond this cookbook, remember that you are not alone. Whether you're just starting out or have been managing Type 2 Diabetes for years, there is a wealth of support and resources available to you. From healthcare professionals who can provide personalized guidance to online communities where you can connect with others on a similar path, know that there is a network of support to help you navigate the challenges and celebrate the victories along the way.

Thank you for allowing me to be a part of your journey toward better health. May your path be filled with nourishing meals, joyful moments, and an abundance of well-being. Here's to your continued success and vitality!

I Have a Request

Have you had the pleasure of diving into the delicious recipes and practical tips within the pages of our Type 2 diabetes cookbook for beginners? We'd love to hear from you!

If you've tried out any of the recipes or simply found inspiration in our cookbook, please consider leaving us a 5 star review. Your feedback is invaluable and helps us continue to improve and provide more of what you love.

Share your thoughts, experiences, and any favorite recipes you've discovered. Your review not only helps us, but also guides fellow cooking enthusiasts in their culinary adventures.

Thank you for being a part of our community! We look forward to hearing from you!

.........*But that's not all! Visit our Author Central page for exclusive content, behind-the-scenes insights, and updates on new releases. Connect with us and join our community of fellow food enthusiasts on a journey to culinary excellence!*

Expand your cookbook collection and elevate your cooking experience with our series. Thank you for your support, and happy cooking! 🍽️✨

UNLOCK YOUR SPECIAL BONUS!!!!!

Scan the Qr Code below to download your free ebook
"Understanding Blood Sugar Level"

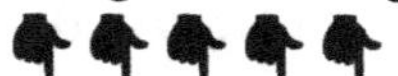